PA

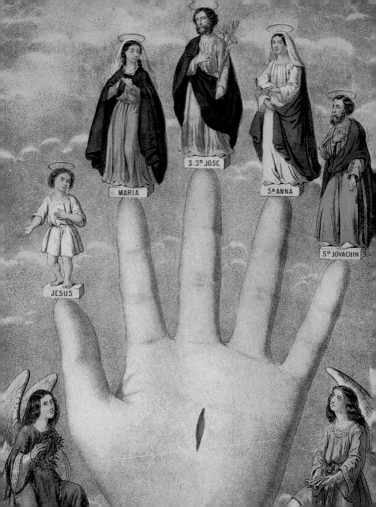

Secrets of

PALM READING

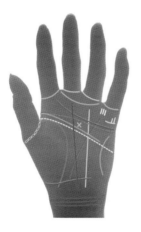

PETER WEST

A Dorling Kindersley Book

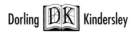

Dorling **DK** Kindersley

LONDON, NEW YORK, SYDNEY, DELHI, PARIS, MUNICH and JOHANNESBURG

First published in The United States of America in 2000 by
DORLING KINDERSLEY PUBLISHING, INC.
95 Madison Avenue, New York, New York 10016

A CIP catalog record for this book is available from the US Library of Congress

ISBN 0-7894-6777-1

This book was conceived, designed and produced by
THE IVY PRESS LIMITED,
The Old Candlemakers,
Lewes, East Sussex BN7 2NZ

Art director *Peter Bridgewater*
Editorial director *Sophie Collins*
Designers *Kevin Knight, Jane Lanaway*
Project Editors *Rowan Davies and Caroline Earle*
Picture researcher *Liz Eddison*
Photography *Guy Ryecart*
Illustrations *Sarah Young, Anna Hunter-Downing*
Three-dimensional models *Mark Jamieson*

Originated and printed by
Hong Kong Graphic and Printing Limited, China

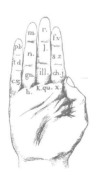

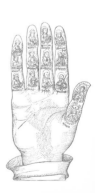

see our complete catalog at

www.dk.com

CONTENTS

How to Use this Book   **6**

Introduction   8

Hand Reading • Understanding the Hands 10

Chiromancy • The Original Palm Reading 62

Practical Palm Reading   **158**

Glossary   218
Further Reading and Useful Addresses   220
Index   222
Acknowledgments   224

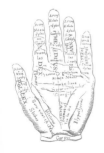
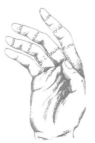
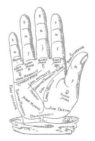

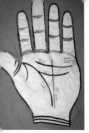

Reading the hands
*The shape of the hand, along with
its lines, mounds, and special
marks, can reveal a great deal
about a person's character.*

HOW TO USE THIS BOOK

To make *Secrets of Palm Reading* easy to use, it has been deliberately split into three distinct sections. The first of these details the basics of hand reading, recognizing the significance of the size and shapes of hand and how to make hand prints suitable for detailed analysis. The second part lists the major and minor lines of the hand along with skin patterns to look out for and their meanings. The third part, *Practical Palm Reading*, shows you how to put what you have learned in the previous sections into practice, along with specially chosen case study examples to follow.

Learning Palm Reading

The aim of this book is to encourage the reader to experiment and to enjoy learning how to develop their hand reading skills. Palm reading today combines modern scientific methods with ancient wisdom, and this book enables the reader to use this knowledge to gain fascinating insights into their own and other people's character traits and life experiences.

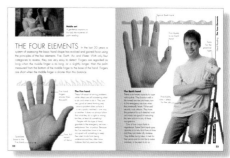

Learning the basics
*The first part gives you the lowdown
on hand shapes and skin patterns.*

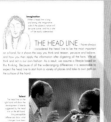

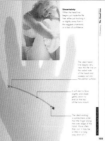

THE HEAD LINE

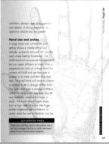

The lines

Practical color spreads show you how to recognize and interpret the meanings of the major and minor lines of the hand.

Detail

Each color section is followed by more detailed information on each aspect of hand reading.

Finger Set

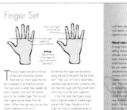

WHICH CAREER?

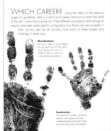

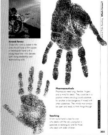

Case studies

Using actual hand print examples you can put all you have learned into practice – you may even be able to tell what the future has in store.

Introduction

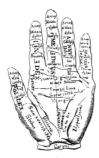

An ancient art
An ancient hand print with Latin inscriptions.

No one can say for certain where palm reading originated. It is possible that it came from the mysterious East, most probably India; or, because it was widely practiced in ancient China, Korea, and Japan, some of its origins can be traced from those countries as well.

Many of the oldest writings and illustrations on palm reading are of Indian origins that seem to predate everything else that we know about. Palm reading was known as long as 5,000 years ago in the Middle East, but not until much later on did the Western world start to record any knowledge of it.

In western Europe and Britain specifically there are a small handful of very rare written records and a few drawings but they are difficult to date. In really ancient times palm reading was largely a superstition; no written rules were set down for anyone to learn, which meant that there was no method or system to be passed along. In those far-off days, few people were able to read and write anyway.

Early English written documentation is sketchy, not so much through a lack of knowledge but rather an inability to set down in writing anything clear-cut. In early Britain before 1066 the official written language was Old English, and even that would have differed dialectically because the country was divided into many kingdoms.

So, what we do know about reading hands was passed down by word of mouth and probably in secret because Mother Church did not approve.

The first printed matter

The oldest known palm reading work in the English language is a manuscript known as the Digby Roll IV, dated around 1440. It is a few strips of vellum sewn together in the style of the time, about 87 inches (220cm) in length and about 8 inches (20cm) in width. A few basic illustrations are included.

The early fortunetellers would have used only the lines when they read the hands of their subjects. Chirognomy was not really developed properly until the middle of the 19th century, and we owe this to two Frenchmen, Casimir D'Arpentigny, who published *La Science de la Main* in 1865, the definitive work on hand shapes, and Adrien Desbarrolles, who published *Les Mystères de la Main* in 1859, based mostly on the study of the lines of the hand. Dermatoglyphics also has its roots in the 19th century and was developed by Francis Galton. From Galton's patient work came the fingerprinting system now used by police in criminal identification.

HAND READING
UNDERSTANDING THE HANDS

Palm reading has managed to remain in the public eye through the centuries despite some quite severe opposition from the established Church. It is known that there are some magnificent old documents to be found in the libraries of the Vatican, but they remain hidden away from general view. ✍ In Britain, during the Dark Ages as the Church fought not only for religious supremacy but also to be a political power, it denounced the practices of astrology and palm reading quite roundly. However, it had to back down where astrology was concerned because there was hardly a medical man who did not use such knowledge before treating patients. ✍ Today, hand analysis may be used as part of a doctor's initial diagnosis as a matter of course.

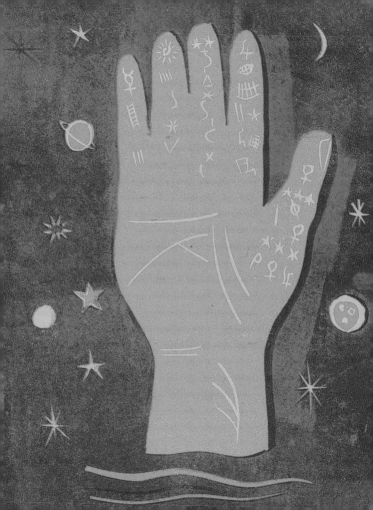

Hand Basics

Hand reading is divided into three quite separate branches that make up the whole study: "chirognomy," the study of the basic shape of the hands; "chiromancy," the study of the lines and other palmar markings; and "dermatoglyphics," the study of the skin patterns found in the fingers and the palmar surface.

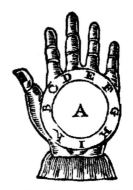

The original palm reading
The frontispiece from Physiognomie and Chiromancie, *one of the earliest printed books on palm reading.*

Chiromancy

This is the study of the lines of the hand without reference to any other feature in the palm. Any of the lines, and especially the smaller influence marks, can change very easily at the time of a serious emotional incident.

When an event such as this occurs and stirs the emotional nature it leaves its mark not only in the psyche but in the hands as well. Minor marks can come and go as and when the heart or mind needs to register such matters because of their importance, at the time or later, when the full import of what has taken place has fully registered. Chiromancy is the original or true palm reading.

Chirognomy

This is the study of the shape of the hand and only really came into its own in the middle of the 19th century. This part of the discipline is concerned with the thickness and shape of the palm, thumb, and fingers, their relative lengths, tip formations, and flexibility. To this has been added a study of the nails and the way the hand may be used in gesture.

Dermatoglyphics

Specifically, this is the study of the fingerprints and the palmar skin patterns. These markings can never be destroyed or erased, but they may be disturbed by accident. There has never been a successful attempt to mutilate or destroy them by the criminal element in an effort to hide them. There are two basic types of palmar patterns: the open, or coarse; and the closed, or refined.

There are five basic skin patterns – the arch, tented arch, composite, loop, and whorl, and to these may be added occasional variations. Each has its own meanings and these are refined dependent on how they appear and where they are formed.

Gesture

It is only in recent times that a study of hand gestures has been added to hand analysis. It is not generally appreciated how much information may be given away by an individual's sign language, either as the person speaks or with small silent movements that can mean so much.

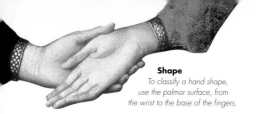

Shape

*To classify a hand shape,
use the palmar surface, from
the wrist to the base of the fingers.*

HAND SHAPES
There are two basic shapes: the square, or useful, and the round, or conic; then there are five other types to consider. Both hands must be carefully examined. We look to the left hand to establish hereditary traits of the personality and character, while the right hand will show how far these tendencies have developed. Even when the subject is left-handed, this holds true.

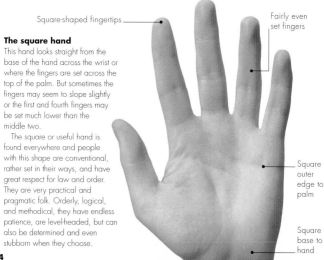

Square-shaped fingertips

Fairly even set fingers

The square hand

This hand looks straight from the base of the hand across the wrist or where the fingers are set across the top of the palm. But sometimes the fingers may seem to slope slightly or the first and fourth fingers may be set much lower than the middle two.

The square or useful hand is found everywhere and people with this shape are conventional, rather set in their ways, and have great respect for law and order. They are very practical and pragmatic folk. Orderly, logical, and methodical, they have endless patience, are level-headed, but can also be determined and even stubborn when they choose.

Square outer edge to palm

Square base to hand

Philosophic hand

Long, bony fingers with a rectangular or square palm are found on this type. Its owners are deep thinkers and take some understanding.

Psychic hand

Narrow, delicate fingers are seen on this extreme version of the conic hand. Psychic hands are beautifully kept, with a long palm.

Mixed hand

All types of finger and palm shapes are found on mixed hands. If what you see cannot be classified, then it is a mixed hand.

Spatulate hand

Fingertips bulge slightly on this variation of the square hand. The palm has a defined widening either at the base or top of the hand.

Elementary hand

Short, stubby fingers classify this type. The whole hand looks short and clumsy with a thick, heavy palm. It suggests limited thinking.

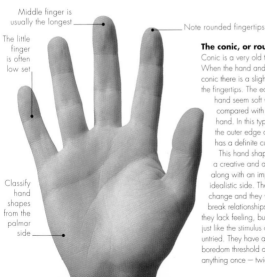

Middle finger is usually the longest

Note rounded fingertips

The little finger is often low set

Classify hand shapes from the palmar side

The conic, or round hand

Conic is a very old term for round. When the hand and fingers are conic there is a slight tapering to the fingertips. The edges of the hand seem soft when compared with a square hand. In this type of hand the outer edge of the palm has a definite curve.

This hand shape indicates a creative and artistic nature, along with an impulsive and idealistic side. These folk like change and they will make and break relationships, not because they lack feeling, but because they just like the stimulus of the new and untried. They have a very low boredom threshold and they will try anything once — twice if they like it!

Hand Size

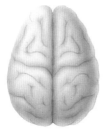

Brain power
*The hand you use more is governed
by the hemispheres of the brain.*

It is most important to remember that
hand size must be assessed in relation
to a person's build. In certain
specialized industries there may be a
proliferation of one type or another.
Large-handed people may be found
working in the jewelry trade, while
small-handed folk are often seen in
practical, creative endeavors such
as selling or advertising.

The large hand

Large hands belong to those who may
be thought superficial rather than
profound, for people with such hands

can fritter away their talent in mindless
attention to detail rather than dealing
with the whole picture. The large hand
generally reflects an analytical mind.

The small hand

People with small hands perceive the
whole picture immediately, but they lack
the appreciation of detail that is needed
to break down the problem into its
component parts. For them it is usually
all or nothing. Small hands with long
palms and short fingers can mean that
detail is given only lip service and is
soon forgotten; memories can be
surprisingly shortlived unless concerned
with matters dear to the owner.

Left- or right-handed?

Right-handedness is directly related
to the development of intelligence in
humankind. The more developed
hemisphere of the brain is usually the left
half and correlates with the right-hand
side of the body. In left-handed folk this
is reversed, although the left hemisphere
may still be the more developed.

Left-handed people to a large extent have to live in a right-handed world and, as a result, their awareness and perception levels are often very highly developed. They will be impatient with long-winded types who take their time to explain matters for left-handers can grasp the essentials of almost anything they take up within a very short space of time. They are then eager to go away and begin their project without any further delay.

Often, others dislike or envy their abilities and left-handers may find it difficult to be accepted.

However, whether left- or right-handed, people with large hands need to have full details of any new project before they start work. Those with small hands can work very well in the background and do not always seek recognition for their work.

The Elements

Hand shapes can also be assessed using the principles of the four elements: Earth, Air, Water, and Fire – see pages 22–29.

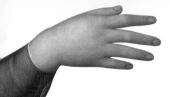

Long or short?

Long fingers mean detail, short fingers see the whole story.

THE BACK OF THE HAND

Casual observation of the back of the hands yields a mine of information especially when traveling – you have a captive set of guinea pigs. People are often at their most relaxed and tend to employ many unconscious gestures. Note how people hold their pens. See if they wear a ring or rings and if so, on which finger or fingers. Check on which wrist they wear their watch or other jewelry and, if they do, whether they favor gold or silver.

The square hand

These folk tend to dress conventionally even on the weekends when most people relax and dress down.

Notice the color of the hands if you can because those with red, square hands enjoy good health and the outdoors. Blue hands suggest they could have circulation problems, while a yellow tinge may imply liver or kidney problems.

It would be rare to see a dead-white square hand for that suggests social apathy carried to an extreme. These folk rarely venture out to meetings or visit friends and neighbors. Normally, they are fairly friendly but do not always encourage intimate relationships.

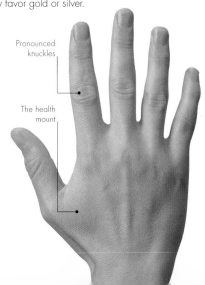

Pronounced knuckles

The health mount

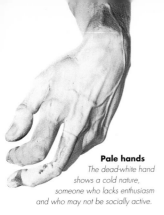

Pale hands
The dead-white hand shows a cold nature, someone who lacks enthusiasm and who may not be socially active.

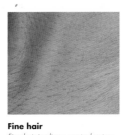

Fine hair
Fine hair implies a genteel nature, one not too physically strong, whereas coarse hair suggests good physical well-being.

The conic hand
People with round hands dress as they see fit and are not always worried about how they look to others. They are more concerned with how they feel in what they are wearing and are rarely over-bothered with convention.

As a rule the conic hand looks pink. This suggests a well-adjusted individual, normally out-going and with plenty of energy. Never averse to burning the candle at both ends, they always enjoy social functions at any level and are emotionally responsive. White conic hands may mean simple anemia or a lowered body temperature through tiredness.

Those with conic hands talk a lot once they feel relaxed but there is little meaning to what they say. Empty chatter to keep an event going is one of the tricks of their trade in making sure everybody has a good time.

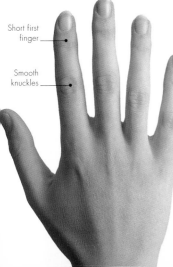

Short first finger

Smooth knuckles

The Back of the Hand

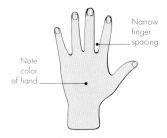

The other side
The back of the hand gives as many clues as the front.

O ften, the first opportunity to look at hands in some detail is to take advantage of someone by observing the backs of the hands. It does pay to make such an appraisal because of the astonishing amount of information that can be gleaned by this exercise.

For example, those with short fingers or small hands want short precise answers, not long or detailed explanations, whereas those with big hands need more detail because they have to weigh up all the possibilities before they take any action.

Length and texture

Long, narrow hands indicate people who take time to think everything through before committing themselves. If the fingers display bulging at each of the phalangeal joints, the capacity for detail is enormous.

When hands are wide across the back this reveals someone who will not stand for any nonsense. Such people are materialists and they like the outdoor life. When the skin looks sunburned or weather-beaten or the texture is rough to the touch, all sorts of outdoor pursuits attract. It may also reflect the craftsperson who prefers to work outdoors, especially if the hand is square shaped.

Narrow, smooth, or pale hands with a soft texture indicate a love of indoor life. If they are lightly tanned in hot sunny weather this shows that the owner may have indulged an innate lazy streak simply by lying out in the sun.

An expanse of skin seen between the end of the nail and the tip of the finger shows a hasty and explosive temper.

In general, those with large nails have a balanced and expansive attitude to life, while small nails show a more critical and restricted approach to life.

Differences

Any obvious differences between two hands are caused mainly by accident or through illness and once seen they are never forgotten. At other times this may refer to someone who has had to fight to maintain a balance in the early family relationship where the parents had quite different personalities. When the hands look more or less the same the subject's inner nature is well balanced.

Such personalities will not encourage too much change in the way that they conduct their personal lives. They generally present themselves in the same manner to all and sundry irrespectively.

Hair on the Hand

Hair on the hand has always been taken to be a sign of a good constitution but not necessarily physical strength – an old belief now proven incorrect.

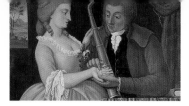

Noble art
A gentleman explains to his lady the mysteries of palm reading.

THE FOUR ELEMENTS
In the last 30 years a system of assessing the basic hand shape has evolved and gained favor using the principles of the four elements: Fire, Earth, Air, and Water. With only four categories to assess, they are very easy to detect. Fingers are regarded as long when the middle finger is as long, or is slightly longer, than the palm measured from the bottom of the middle finger to the base of the hand. Fingers are short when the middle finger is shorter than this distance.

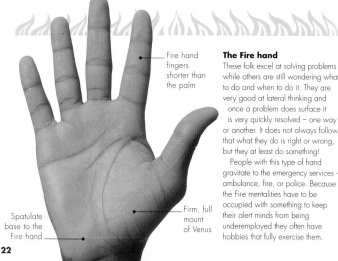

Fire hand fingers shorter than the palm

Spatulate base to the Fire hand

Firm, full mount of Venus

The Fire hand
These folk excel at solving problems while others are still wondering what to do and when to do it. They are very good at lateral thinking and once a problem does surface it is very quickly resolved – one way or another. It does not always follow that what they do is right or wrong, but they at least do something!

People with this type of hand gravitate to the emergency services – ambulance, fire, or police. Because the Fire mentalities have to be occupied with something to keep their alert minds from being underemployed they often have hobbies that fully exercise them.

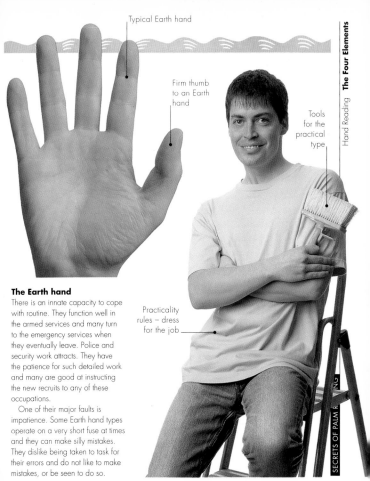

Typical Earth hand

Firm thumb to an Earth hand

Tools for the practical type

The Earth hand

There is an innate capacity to cope with routine. They function well in the armed services and many turn to the emergency services when they eventually leave. Police and security work attracts. They have the patience for such detailed work and many are good at instructing the new recruits to any of these occupations.

One of their major faults is impatience. Some Earth hand types operate on a very short fuse at times and they can make silly mistakes. They dislike being taken to task for their errors and do not like to make mistakes, or be seen to do so.

Practicality rules – dress for the job

Fire and Earth Hands

The Fire hand

This hand has a rectangular palm with fingers shorter than the palm. In many cases the fingers may seem to be a trifle wider at their tips. This shape implies an extrovert nature, for these folk are bright and intelligent and have natural leadership talents, always able to take charge when others fail.

Because they are also so mentally alive they flourish best when organizing others and getting things done. Man-management is second nature; they inspire and motivate others with their natural zeal.

Fire sign folk have a lazy streak and, with many, there is an in-built self-destruct mode. They cannot always manage whatever natural reserves they have, and many have been known to burn themselves out.

They need a diligent second-in-command who can take charge of the basic routine work and stop things from going wrong before it is too late. They acknowledge these assistants are needed in such circumstances.

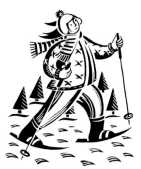

Taking it to extremes
Any sport that really taxes both the mind and body always attracts Fire hand types.

Fire hand people are best suited to occupations that keep them on the move or are full of change and variety. The selling game is ideal for them, especially when it involves demonstrations of the product.

Sports attract, and so does the entertainment world, for both are natural outlets for these exhibitionists – but they run the risk of burning themselves out too soon. Because they have such a love of change and variety these extroverts might enjoy politics.

The Earth hand

People with a square palm and slightly shorter fingers are down-to-earth, reliable, and conventional folk. They are at their best when maintaining law and order and will not stand for any nonsense. Personal discipline is a must; they must present an air of authority and calm at all times.

Very strong on tradition, they will not break the rules or even bend them to achieve an aim. They are always neat and tidy with a place for everything and with everything in its place. They do well in outdoor occupations, such as gardening, farming, or building, and they also work very well with animals.

When there is a distinct curve or bulge running down the outer edge of the palm it indicates very strong creative abilities and leanings. These people normally possess great manual dexterity.

Short Fuses

Earth hand types can make you feel very small when they throw the book at you – so heaven help you if you make a mistake!

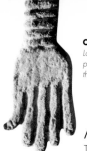

Creative minds
Long, thin fingers and bony palms are characteristic of the creative Air hand types.

AIR AND WATER HANDS

These people are not always able to keep their feet on the ground as much as the Fire and Earth types. Air folk tend to have their heads in the clouds thinking things through, while the Water types become easily caught up with their strong imagination. The creativity of the minds of Air and Water people often carries them away at the drop of hat.

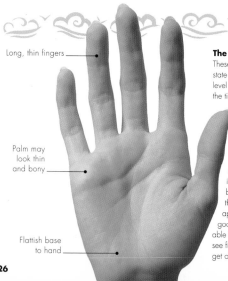

Long, thin fingers

Palm may look thin and bony

Flattish base to hand

The Air hand

These folk prefer to be in a constant state of intellectual stimulation at any level or whatever suits them the best at the time, for their moods can fluctuate wildly. Their companions will be important to them; they like to be sure their friends operate on a similar comparative level.

Communication is important; it has to be right and suit the subject at hand. If the mood is light, they thrive on a gentle banter. If the tone is serious, they match it with a suitable approach. They are often very good at initiating ideas and are able to persuade and cajole as they see fit to ensure their pet projects get off the ground.

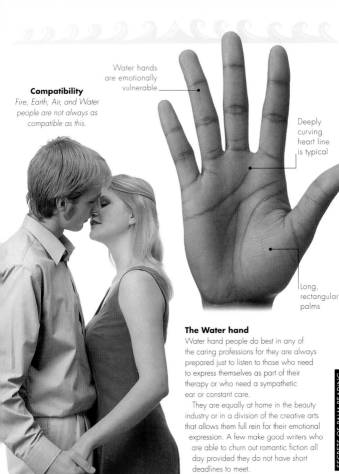

Water hands are emotionally vulnerable

Deeply curving heart line is typical

Long, rectangular palms

Compatibility

Fire, Earth, Air, and Water people are not always as compatible as this.

The Water hand

Water hand people do best in any of the caring professions for they are always prepared just to listen to those who need to express themselves as part of their therapy or who need a sympathetic ear or constant care.

They are equally at home in the beauty industry or in a division of the creative arts that allows them full rein for their emotional expression. A few make good writers who are able to churn out romantic fiction all day provided they do not have short deadlines to meet.

Air and Water Hands

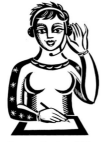

Communication skills
*A typical Air hand occupation could
be a telephonist/receptionist.*

The Air hand

The typical Air hand has a square palm with fingers longer than the palm and is often flexible and supple. Well-balanced and reliable folk, Air hand people are very creative and crave variety in just about all they do. They must be kept busy, for then they are at their very best!

Air hand types are socially gifted and thrive in company. However, while they are popular, in emotional relationships they can seem to be somewhat controlled – almost as if they are scared to "let go." They often find it difficult to express themselves emotionally and are not given to impulsive behavior of any kind.

While they appear to learn from their experiences, they seem unable to cope with one-to-one relationships and issues. As a result their private lives are very changeable. Too much time is spent controlling their responses; they tackle problems with excessive logic.

Air hands thrive in the communications field. There is a flair for languages and an understanding of modern technology such as computers and the Internet. If it involves communication, then Air hand types are happy to play.

The entertainment industry is alive with Air hands because they have mercurial minds and an unflappable attitude. Many actors with Air hand characteristics often look to working behind the camera and turn into excellent directors, and soon learn how to be producers, because they can turn disadvantage into advantage with ease. They also know how to make, and keep, money.

The Water hand

Long rectangular palms with rather long and graceful fingers typify the warm emotional nature of the Water hand. In fact, these people are more emotionally orientated than is good for them; their moods can swing in either direction so easily that it is difficult to know what they will do next or how they will react.

The circumstances have to be just right if you want to get the best out of Water hand people. They are fluid, changeable, and impressionable, and often unreliable because they think with their hearts rather than with their minds.

So, they need to learn to keep both feet very firmly on the ground at all times. When a new romance starts, a frequent event in their lives, it sends them into a world totally of their own making. They probably fall in love with love rather the object of their affections.

Sensitive Types

Water hands, also known as sensitive hands, are vulnerable individuals who are not well suited to the pressures of the modern world.

FINGERS

The shape and development of the fingers individually and collectively relate to the instinctive side of personality and character, whereas the palm represents the practical side of the subject's nature. Fingers must be examined from all sides, and the fingers of both hands must be compared with each other. It is important to assess their relationship not only to one another but also to other parts of the hand. The tips are classified differently and will be dealt with later.

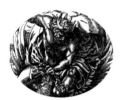

Jupiter

Jupiter is associated with knowledge and learning, and was assigned to the index finger.

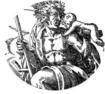

Saturn

Associated with balance, restriction, and caution, Saturn was assigned to the middle finger.

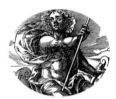

Apollo

Apollo implies creativity and general joie de vivre, and was given rulership of the third finger.

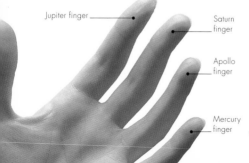

Jupiter finger

Saturn finger

Apollo finger

Mercury finger

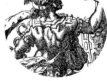

Mercury

Mercury, messenger of the gods, was assigned to the little finger, for it speaks volumes in gesture.

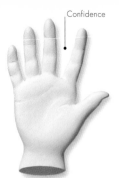

Confidence

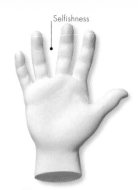

Selfishness

First and second fingers

When there is a wide space between the first and second fingers there is a sense of inner confidence and independence. This type is a leader.

Middle and ring fingers

A wide space between the middle and ring fingers shows a resourceful and selfish nature, one who may not always think of others when making decisions.

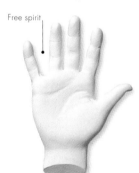

Free spirit

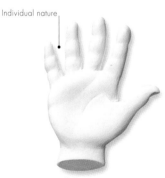

Individual nature

Third and fourth fingers

Wide spacing between the third and fourth fingers indicates a lone wolf type who needs to be as free as the air. They dislike wasting energy or time.

All fingers

Wide spacing between all of the fingers means the subject is inclined to be an extrovert, for such people prize their individuality and freedom of thought.

Length and Appearance

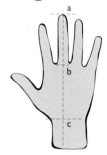

Finger length
*Measure the middle finger against
the palm to assess length.*

To establish whether fingers are
long or short, take a ruler and
measure the middle finger from its
tip (a) to the crease where it joins the
top of the palm (b). Measure from this
point to the bottom of the palm where
the skin pattern fades out (c).

If the middle finger is shorter than the
palm, then the fingers are all classified
as short. When it is longer than the
palm, the fingers should all be classified
as long. It is quite rare for the middle
finger to be shorter than the others but
when this is the case measure the
longest finger instead.

Smooth fingers

When fingers appear smooth, that is,
without any indication of bulging or
knotting at the joints, the owner is
perceptive, versatile, and intuitive. If the
fingers are short, impulsiveness is strong.

Those with long, smooth fingers
thrive on intricate and detailed work
and stop to review matters at the
appropriate times.

Knotted fingers

Knotting or bulging at the phalangeal
joints acts as a check on the inward flow
of information. If found on each finger joint
it indicates a very critical nature.

Knots at the top joint imply slow-to-
please types who try to "cross their
bridges" before they come to them.
Pronounced lower joints show a
pragmatic and methodical type.

The knuckles

When the knuckles are all reasonably
even, the subjects will have a way of
always looking neat and tidy no
matter what they wear. They may be

concerned with diet, fitness, and personal discipline. People with uneven knuckles present an outward appearance of being tidy, but it is only superficial. Their homes may look neat and tidy but if you open a drawer or lift a cushion their real character will be shown with all its deficiencies.

Each finger should be examined carefully phalange by phalange. Check for knotting or a pronounced bulge at each phalangeal joint and at the knuckles. Take the time to assess each finger against its neighbor and note any obvious disparity.

After this, check the fingers of each hand against its partner on the other hand. There are nearly always slight changes to be observed and these little points help to account for those quirks of personality not always immediately apparent when you first look.

The Thumb

For information on interpreting the significance of the length and shape of the thumb, see pages 38–41.

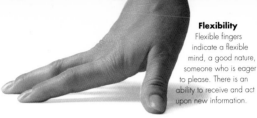

Flexibility
Flexible fingers
indicate a flexible
mind, a good nature,
someone who is eager
to please. There is an
ability to receive and act
upon new information.

FLEXIBILITY AND NAIL TYPES

The flexibility of the hand reflects that person's character: a flexible hand indicates a flexible mind, while a stiff hand shows a stubborn or unyielding nature. The open hand shows an open mind while a closed hand suggests small-mindedness and a tendency to be critical. It is also important to look at the subject's nails during a hand reading; they will give you vital clues to the person's health and lifestyle.

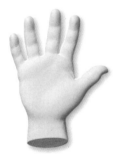

confidence and this type is a follower, rather than a leader.

A narrow space between the second and third fingers suggests the subject is always thinking of the immediate and distant future.

When there is a narrow gap between the third and fourth fingers there is always a lot of dependency on others, for such people believe in safety in numbers.

If all the spaces between the fingers are narrow, the person's nature is closed, subjective, and very dependent on what others think. In this case the subject's initiative levels will be low.

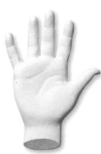

Narrow spaces
Spacing between the fingers is either narrow or wide. When the space between the first and middle fingers is narrow the owner prefers to go along with the crowd; there is a lack of

Inflexibility
With stiff or unyielding fingers there will be an accompanying stiff and unyielding nature and a selfish streak thrown in. This type tends to be somewhat conservative and conventional.

Almond nail
This type implies a steady and refined character and personality. People with almond nails make loyal, honest, and truthful friends.

Shell-shaped nail
This nail indicates poor health and ultra-sensitivity along with the rundown state that follows a shock to the system.

Talon-shaped nail
This type of nail shows generally poor diet-consciousness, which in turn will affect the owner's state of health.

Square nail
The short square-shaped nail always indicates a basically critical nature. Such folk lack real warmth and depth of feeling.

Healthy nail
The nails are a great indicator of a person's health and lifestyle. Check your nails regularly for telltale signs.

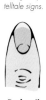

Red nail
Nails with a reddish hue indicate a hot-tempered individual.

Check for ridging or fluting

Note the color of the nail

Look for white flecks

Half moons should be visible

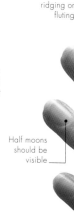

Nail shapes
There are four basic nail shapes, but in practice there may be as many as ten.

Finger Set

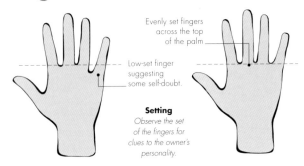

Evenly set fingers across the top of the palm

Low-set finger suggesting some self-doubt.

Setting
Observe the set of the fingers for clues to the owner's personality.

The way fingers are set on the top of the palm should be noticed; there are four main types that can be compared to architectural arches. The most usual is when they appear set like a Norman arch with the central point at the middle finger. The first and little fingers are set lower than the others. When they are very low set they make a perpendicular arch.

A low-set first finger always signifies a lack of self-confidence; the lower it is, the less "push" there will be in the personality. When the little finger is set low expect to find an inferiority complex of some degree or another. There is always some element of self-doubt.

Sometimes the fingers are set evenly along the top of the palm like the Tudor arch. Here, you will find a reasonably well-balanced personality, someone who can take the rough with the smooth and who trusts his or her own judgment.

In the final type, the fingers slope from a high-set index to a seemingly low-set little finger. People with this finger set have a misplaced sense of self-confidence; they bluff their way through life until they are found out.

When you assess the finger settings you must always take into account the overall appearance of the hand itself. A large open hand, wide spacing, and evenly set fingers suggest the nature is confident, always open to suggestion and reason. A strong degree of co-operation should also be present.

Hand size and arches

A large hand with a Norman arch setting shows a middle-of-the-road attitude, someone who will not rock the boat unless feeling threatened. The small hand will accentuate this approach but can seem diffident at times. With a perpendicular arch on a large hand the owners will bluff and use their size to appear a lot more confident than they feel. The small hand will have to scheme to appear to be in charge of their lives. The Tudor arch type is always confident, and if the hand is stiff they may also be very stubborn, whether it is large or small. The hand where fingers slope from a high index to a low little finger exhibit misplaced self-confidence no matter what the size or flexibility may be.

Sensitivity Pads

These are small fleshy pads on the palmar side of the first phalanges that show a highly developed sense of touch and emotional extremes.

THE THUMB

This has always been considered to be the most important part of hand analysis, and for centuries it has been known as the signature of the hand and is a major key in the assessment of character. On any pair of hands no two thumbs are ever really alike; there will always be a slight difference. These differences must be taken into account especially when there is a wide disparity between the hands anyway.

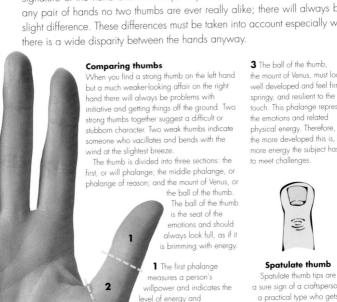

Comparing thumbs

When you find a strong thumb on the left hand but a much weaker-looking affair on the right hand there will always be problems with initiative and getting things off the ground. Two strong thumbs together suggest a difficult or stubborn character. Two weak thumbs indicate someone who vacillates and bends with the wind at the slightest breeze.

The thumb is divided into three sections: the first, or will phalange; the middle phalange, or phalange of reason; and the mount of Venus, or the ball of the thumb. The ball of the thumb is the seat of the emotions and should always look full, as if it is brimming with energy.

1 The first phalange measures a person's willpower and indicates the level of energy and decisiveness.

2 The middle phalange shows how a subject reasons things through before deciding on the path they should take.

3 The ball of the thumb, the mount of Venus, must look well developed and feel firm, springy, and resilient to the touch. This phalange represents the emotions and related physical energy. Therefore, the more developed this is, the more energy the subject has to meet challenges.

Spatulate thumb

Spatulate thumb tips are a sure sign of a craftsperson, a practical type who gets things done. However, these people are all too ready to pursue the attraction of the moment and will drop whatever they are doing for anything new and untried.

The spokeshave thumb tip tapers toward the top and is best seen from the side, and it denotes great powers of persuasion

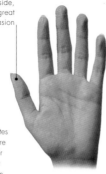

Pointed thumb

A pointed thumb tip indicates an idealist, people who are very clever at getting their own way. They are very persuasive and there is an in-built knack for spotting the weakness of others and seizing advantage. If the tip is soft to the touch, then the nature is inclined to be more submissive.

Low-set thumb

The lower the thumb on the side of the hand, the more inspirational the character. If wide angled, an adventurer; if narrow, conventional.

High-set thumb

A thumb high up on the hand, a long way from the wrist, suggests a good and clearly defined instinctive creative flair.

Square-tipped thumb

A square tip suggests a realist and a hard taskmaster but one who will lead by example. There is a strong sense of fair play and justice. These people may seem hard or unfeeling when they are in a position of leadership.

Conic tip

People with a conic or round tip on their thumbs respond far too readily to external stimuli and are easily distracted. While these folk may be quick-thinking and sensitive, they are not always as committed as they may first appear.

Bulbous thumb

A bulbous thumb, the old-fashioned "murderer's thumb," shows a strongly physical approach to life with strong appetites. The expression, "resistance is futile," is very apt here, for these people have quite heated tempers.

Length and Angle

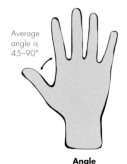

Average angle is 45–90°

Angle
A narrow angle implies caution.
A wide angle suggests generosity.

The length of the thumb should be about equal to the little finger or, when held close to the index finger it ought to be able to reach at least halfway up the third phalange of that finger. When it is relaxed and held naturally, the angle between it and the first finger should be at least 45° to 90°.

The narrower the angle, the more small-minded, prejudiced, and limited the nature. An angle greater than 90° shows resolution and the ability to lead. When the thumb aligns with the fingers in such a way that almost all of the nail can be seen, the nature will be spontaneous and enthusiastic. When the thumb opposes the fingers or stands at right angles to them it is a sign of great self-control. These people are difficult to get to know intimately.

Length of thumb phalanges
A long but well-proportioned thumb shows good personal self-control with a sound ability to take command. If it is overlong, the nature will be stubborn and very determined.

The longer the first phalange the more determined the nature, and a very long first phalange implies a tyrannical nature, while a short first phalange suggests poor leadership abilities.

A short middle phalange reveals poor rational perception and such folk operate best on an intuitive basis. If it is short and thin, the owner flourishes if directed but only within familiar set routines. The longer the middle phalange is, the more these folk must reason everything out before taking the appropriate action.

The short but thick phalange shows the owner lacks tact and diplomacy, while a long thin section implies a logical turn of mind but with a tendency to become embroiled in more detail than is necessary. Those who have the waisted phalange (with concave sides) possess charm, tact, and diplomacy.

If the ball of the thumb greatly outweighs the others, the physical appetites will be very strong. When it appears to be dull there will be little zest or enthusiasm in the personality. The thumb should always look as if it belongs to the hand. It should not appear too large or cumbersome, nor seem to be weak or ineffectual.

Traditionally, the thumb has always been known as the signature of the hand. Whenever you see one that does not appear to belong to the hand then you must interpret it accordingly.

Flexibility

A flexible thumb tip shows an impulsive, easygoing nature. A stiff tip indicates a strict disciplinarian, one who won't compromise.

Francis Galton

A profile of Francis Galton, the father of the modern fingerprint system.

FINGERPRINTS

All human palms, fingers, and the fingertips especially have a fine covering of tiny ridges and furrows called capillary lines that fall into recognized patterns now used mainly to identify people in criminal investigations. In palm reading, they are associated with character and personality. There are similar patterns to be found on the soles of the feet and toes. The markings form in the womb and never change; long after death they may be the only way to identify a body.

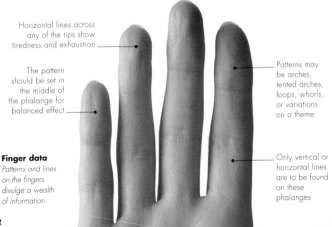

Horizontal lines across any of the tips show tiredness and exhaustion

The pattern should be set in the middle of the phalange for balanced effect

Finger data
Patterns and lines on the fingers divulge a wealth of information.

Patterns may be arches, tented arches, loops, whorls, or variations on a theme

Only vertical or horizontal lines are to be found on these phalanges

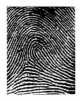

The loop

The loop pattern suggests emotional elasticity. The nature is generally flexible and cooperative.

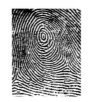

The whorl

The whorl suggests a closed character, one who is not too open. These people are always cool under fire.

The tented arch

Those with a tented arch are born idealists, many of whom strive for a perfect world and who do not like criticism.

The arch

The arch pattern indicates the salt of the Earth personality. These folk are useful, conventional and honest.

The composite

This may be made up of any variation of an arch, a tented arch, or loop with a whorl.

The variation

Variations can occur on one or two fingers. They are best read as composites.

The bigger picture

Use a magnifying glass to observe closely the skin patterns on your hand.

Fingerprint Patterns

I t is vital to remember that we are discussing these patterns in a chirological context and not a criminal investigation, for which the classification is much more complex. In palm reading, we consider three basic fingerprint patterns: the arch, the loop, and the whorl.

Unique
Each fingerprint has a unique pattern.

The arch

The arch pattern looks like a small humpback bridge and suggests a capable and reliable person, someone who can be trusted and who copes well, especially if things go awry. Such people make good, trustworthy friends and reliable employees.

The tented arch

This often looks like a tall loop straight up the phalange. Tented arches imply enthusiasm for life; these people are idealists and reformers and they love change or anything new. They can flatter well and when they want something they know how to get it.

The loop

There are two types of loops: the ulnar and radial. The ulnar loop throws its lariat from the outer edge of the palm, while the radial loop begins at the thumb side of the hand, makes its pattern, and returns. The loop always indicates flexibility and adaptability.

Those with the ulnar loop act instinctively and need to know when to get started; more followers than leaders, for they yield quickly under pressure. The radial loop person is just as flexible, but they have more of a backbone than others. They can resist pressure and are slightly more ambitious and will lead if necessary.

The whorl

The whorl almost always reveals an inflexible nature, individualists who must experience things for themselves. Their character seems cold and unapproachable or they may just find it difficult to open up to others. However,

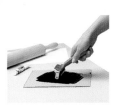

1 *Squeeze out ⅛ inch (¾cm) ink onto the glass plate and roll it out thoroughly until any lumps in the ink have gone.*

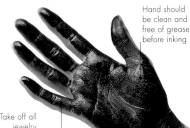

Hand should be clean and free of grease before inking

Take off all jewelry and watches

Include a little of the wrist and the rascettes

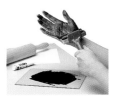

2 *Ink the roller sparingly and ink the hands and the inside of the wrist. Put a sheet of paper on the rolling pin.*

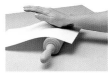

3 *Place the wrist at the bottom of the paper and roll the inked hand back over the rolling pin toward you.*

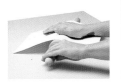

4 *While rolling, make sure that you keep an even pressure so that both the fingertips and thumb are printed.*

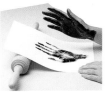

5 *Always lift the hand from the paper, never the other way around for the print may smudge. It will dry within a few moments.*

Whenever you make prints, mark them "left" or "right" as you go and on the back of the print write the details you want to record. As a rule, you will want to record a description of the back of a hand, details of the nails, flexibility, knotting, and other special marks.

For a very quick appraisal, dust the hands lightly with talcum powder and then gently rub them together; the surface marking will be thrown into a fairly clear relief.

Reading Hand Prints

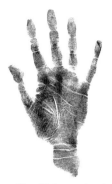

Your life in your hand
*Hand prints record far more
than just the lines.*

Interviews do not always last long or may be conducted in several sessions. You cannot always remember everything afterward, so it makes sense to keep records, and prints are always there for you as valuable reference material. It does not matter how often you look at hand prints, you always find something that you have missed earlier. When interviewing someone over a long period of time, prints taken will record any changes very clearly.

Each print is a negative of the actual hand, so the white lines are the lines of the hands and if the thumb is on the right-hand side then it is a copy of the left hand and vice versa.

If a print is of a satisfactory standard, you should be able to read the fingerprints and the palmar capillary lines, preferably with the naked eye. However, if they can be read clearly under a reasonably powerful magnifying glass that will be fine.

Life-changing experiences

It is very rare for the hand actually to change from one shape to another. I have seen a square hand become softer and more rounded over a period of time and the reverse has also occurred, but it is very unusual. There are a few other recorded instances of such changes referred to by palmists over the years but these are very few and far between.

However, all the lines can and do change according to the type of incident that the owner experiences. If an event is serious enough to leave its mark on the psyche and in the memory of the subject then the palm will record it.

It is here that hand prints prove to be of real value. If a palmist has long-term clients he or she should have taken copies on a regular basis. At first, only occasional changes may be observed but, in the event of a messy divorce or a tragic death, the major lines will change. However, what may seem minor to us may have a devastating effect on someone else. Think of how inwardly sensitive you really are and you will begin to realize how sensitive other people may feel on certain issues.

When advising young people of possible career paths the fate line will record the success or failure from within that individual, and the lines will also show excessive parental pressures.

Thumb Prints

Thumb prints should be made separately by putting the paper at the edge of the table. Put the thumb tip on the bottom and roll it in one direction only or it too will smudge.

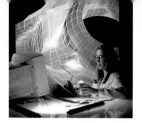

Creative
Those people with an apex on the center of the Apollo mount are practical types with creative flair.

PALMAR SKIN PATTERNS

The skin ridge compositions on the palmar surface, the capillary lines and furrows similar to the designs on the fingertips, form a variety of different patterns that have been found to represent certain facets of character and personality. Each of the mounts under the fingers has a traceable central point – the apex – the meeting point of the ridges and furrows within the skin pattern, known in dermatoglyphics as a tri-radius. We use these central points to measure behavior patterns. Mounts may share the space beneath the fingers, forming one extra large mound, and central points will incline one way or the other.

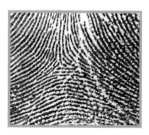

Locating the apex
To locate the central point, trace the series of ridges and furrows where they meet in a triangular formation. The apex is the meeting point of the ridges and furrows within the skin pattern.

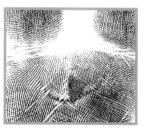

Locating apices on the mounts
When the apex is more under the first finger than the middle, read it as a Jupiter/Saturn mount; if it is more under the middle finger, read it as a Saturn/Jupiter mount. Use this idea for other pairings.

Open and Closed Patterns

There are two distinct types of skin patterns: closed or smooth, and rough or open. When the pattern appears closed or fine, the nature is gentle and somewhat refined. These people are persuasive and perceptive. The open pattern shows wide furrows and ridges that are seen in the hands of the physically active. They indicate a materialist and practical outlook.

Apices on the mounts

Each digital mount has an apex in the skin pattern that is used to establish the center of that mount.

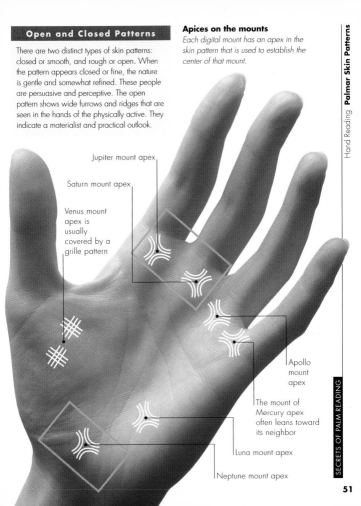

Jupiter mount apex

Saturn mount apex

Venus mount apex is usually covered by a grille pattern

Apollo mount apex

The mount of Mercury apex often leans toward its neighbor

Luna mount apex

Neptune mount apex

The Apices on the Mounts

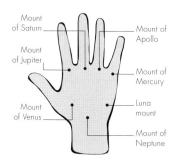

Mount of Saturn
Mount of Jupiter
Mount of Venus
Mount of Apollo
Mount of Mercury
Luna mount
Mount of Neptune

The mounts
Fleshy prominences under the fingers and on the palm are known as mounts.

The mount of Jupiter

A central apex indicates integrity, pride, and responsibility. If it leans toward the thumb there is an aversion to red tape, when toward the medius, the subject respects law and order.

The mount of Saturn

This apex is often high set and inclines to the first finger or the third. It shows a practical approach. If it leans toward the Jupiter finger the owner may have a collecting hobby, while if toward the Apollo the subject is more sociable.

The mount of Apollo

A centrally placed apex shows a practical and artistic nature. If it inclines toward the medius, the subject will find it hard to trust people and may be inhibited. When it leans toward the Mercury mount there will be a talent for salesmanship and for making and losing money. Sometimes, the rules may be broken and fraud may result.

The mount of Mercury

This apex is rarely centrally placed and almost always leans inward, but when the apex is placed centrally under the little finger it helps the subject's popularity. When it is directly under the fourth finger there is a talent for communications. If placed nearer the percussion – the outer edge of the hand – these gifts are enhanced.

The Luna mount

If there is a tri-radius it will act as a line between the Luna mount and Venus, generally more toward the Luna mount. The lower it is the less it seems to affect anything, but a high-set apex may show weakness of the cardiovascular system. If the fate line passes through the triradius, career matters never seem quite to get started. When the sun line makes a path through the pattern, hopes and wishes may come to nothing.

The mount of Venus

This apex is usually hidden by the grille formation but occasionally one may be seen. If in the middle of the mount it shows a good constitution and libido. If placed low, basic instincts rule, while a high-set apex implies prudishness.

The mount of Neptune

An apex here exerts little influence on its own, but when the fate line starts here or the life line ends here or passes through, the owner may lean toward astrology, palm reading, or similar practices.

The Mounts

For more details on all the mounts and their meanings see pages 74–77.

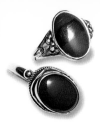

Rings on their fingers
*Rings emphasize the
meaning of the finger
on which they are worn.*

RINGS AND THINGS
Palm reading is not just looking at a hand and interpreting what is found there. You must look at the whole picture. If a watch is worn, note how and on which wrist, for this always helps you in the overall assessment. A watch on the left wrist is the norm, while one on the right suggests the owner might be fussy, left-handed, ambidextrous, or a poseur. If it is worn under the wrist, they might be sportspeople or outdoor workers and are simply protecting it. But rings have a very different set of meanings.

Watches
*Analogue watches imply a
traditional approach; digital
ones are more modern.*

Middle finger
accentuates
a feeling
of balance —————

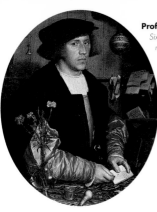

Professional adornment

Sixteenth-century merchants wore a ring on the first finger, an indication of their professional status.

GOLD   SILVER

Good and evil

Wear gold during daylight hours and silver during the night. Gold is the metal of the sun and all things that are truly righteous. Silver is the metal of the witches, of the dark forces, and those who might deceive.

A ring here suggests a desire for independence

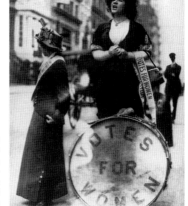

Women's rights

In the 19th century a ring worn on a woman's little finger often indicated an independent spirit and support for the women's rights movement.

The Significance of Rings

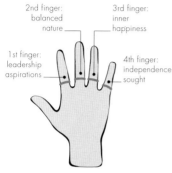

2nd finger:
balanced
nature

3rd finger:
inner
happiness

1st finger:
leadership
aspirations

4th finger:
independence
sought

Which finger?

*The finger on which a ring is worn
indicates certain personality traits.*

Very often, a ring and how and on which finger it is worn can suggest that the owner is ignorant of any message. However, these messages have been passed down to us from the 16th century when there were precise meanings. A doctor wore his ring on his thumb; merchants or businessmen wore one on the first finger. Those who put a ring on the middle finger were thought to be of poor intelligence. Students would wear rings on the third finger.

Lovers irrespective of their age would wear a ring on the fourth finger. In England, during the reign of George I very heavy wedding rings were worn on the thumb. But these days they are worn on the third finger of the left hand because it was believed a special nerve or vein led from there directly to the heart. In most of Europe, women prefer the right hand.

Rings were not always worn at the base of a finger; some used to be worn on the middle phalange. A special affectation was shown when a ring was worn on the nail phalange.

Rings and personality

Rings are traditionally believed to enhance or emphasize the qualities of the finger on which they are worn. On the first finger, therefore, they imply leadership qualities.

A ring on the middle finger suggests a cold nature, people well aware but unsure of their own emotional vulnerability. Inwardly lonely, it is difficult for them to open up socially.

Most people wear a ring on the third finger as a matter of course. Allegedly, it indicates a fondness for social affairs but also shows that these people don't like being on their own for too long. This is the traditional finger with which to indicate their married or single status.

Little finger rings may relate many messages. Freemasons wear a ring here, often obvious from the design that traces back to the "surprise ring" of the 17th century. It had a hinged surface that would reveal a magical or other marking indicating membership of a secret group or sect.

In the 19th century, a ring worn here by a woman showed allegiance to women's rights movements and her newly independent character. These women often had their portraits painted with a ring conspicuously on this finger.

Thumb Rings

These are now being seen again, but they are very uncomfortable to wear. This is a fashion statement that implies the owner wants to be seen to be different.

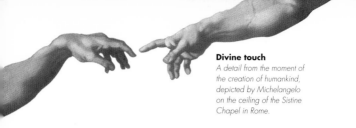

Divine touch
A detail from the moment of the creation of humankind, depicted by Michelangelo on the ceiling of the Sistine Chapel in Rome.

HAND GESTURES
We exhibit a part of our real nature in our daily contact with everyone we meet. As we talk, our hands help to accentuate some of the points we want to make. We learn this as a matter of course from a very early age because we constantly mimic our elders as we grow up. When with other people, we listen, observe, and recognize characteristics that we associate with those people, but half the time we do not do this consciously – it's all performed without thinking about it. However, whatever a hand gesture may prove or disprove, you must remember that it is not universal.

Ambiguous
What might mean one thing in one country can and does often mean something entirely different in another.

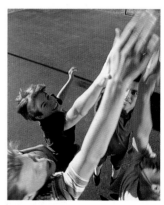

High five
Hand gestures accentuate the spoken word. The "high five" is a gesture of greeting or mutual congratulation in many countries.

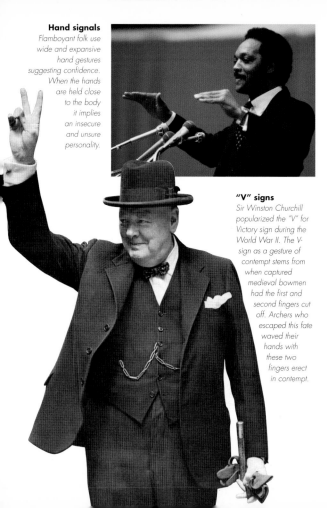

Hand signals

Flamboyant folk use wide and expansive hand gestures suggesting confidence. When the hands are held close to the body it implies an insecure and unsure personality.

"V" signs

Sir Winston Churchill popularized the "V" for Victory sign during the World War II. The V-sign as a gesture of contempt stems from when captured medieval bowmen had the first and second fingers cut off. Archers who escaped this fate waved their hands with these two fingers erect in contempt.

Interpreting Hand Gestures

I had a dream my life would be . . .

Ich träumte mein Leben wäre . . .

Tenía un sueño en el que mi . . .

Handwriting
*The handwriting style can
reflect the type of hand.*

Handwriting is a silent but observable result of consistent gestures, shaped intelligence, and the emotional state of the writer at the time. In fact, handwriting is such a personal natural movement it cannot really be disguised. Would-be palmists should study the basic techniques of handwriting to help their analyses.

Handshakes

A handshake implies good will, but the act itself varies quite a lot and some people will not offer their hand, preferring to just nod or smile. This is a sign of a closed personality – deliberate and conscious control. A person may hold the hand palm down or in the dominant position, because this will make the other person turn the hand palm upward in a gesture of submission.

The powerhouse handshake, when your hand is seized, squeezed, or pumped and thrown back, shows insecurity covered by a mask of a pseudo-macho personality – a bluffer.

If the offered hand is awkward to hold so that you have to do the work, you may feel superior, exactly what the other person wants. They are clever, designing, and deceptive, bluffing others into a false sense of security.

The type who pumps your hand and touches your shoulder with a feigned gesture of intimacy is off-putting. They are full of false promises.

Silent signals

The forefinger with an accompanying clenched fist is emphatic and quite unmistakable in its meaning. The other hand will show you how controlled the person is. If it is held open, the point is made. If closed, prepare for potential physical aggression. Think for a moment, while the first finger accuses, the others are all tucked up in their fist, pointing at themselves, virtually saying that some of the blame is theirs.

People who hold the hands open but with their backs toward you pleading innocence are probably not. If they show you their open palms, they may well be telling the truth. Hiding the palm implies hiding the true self, while showing the palm reveals an open nature and an honest person.

Arms that are crossed over the chest indicate defensiveness; if the hands hold the arms, then pride is hurt, but if they just rest on the arms, problems will be easier to resolve. A hand raised to the throat signifies insecurity and probably imminent capitulation. Frequently, there is a slight lowering of the head at the same time, showing that you have won.

Open or Closed?

Hand gestures should be open. When they are closed the owner is not being "open" with you; closed hands show possible deception.

CHIROMANCY
THE ORIGINAL PALM READING

While still in the womb, the principal lines of life, head, and heart and a couple of others, perhaps, can be seen at as early as four months; the rest begin to show a little later. 🐌 Unlike the skin patterns that never change, these lines can and do vary according to the experiences of the individual. As youngsters mature, the strengths and weaknesses of character and personality can affect the way the lines are reflected in the palm if certain incidents have registered sufficiently within their psyches. 🐌 In ancient times only the lines were interpreted; analysis of shape and other features came much later. The palm indicates the general nature, while the lines show how this is put to use, for good or ill. Always remember to check both hands very carefully, for any differences can affect the overall assessment.

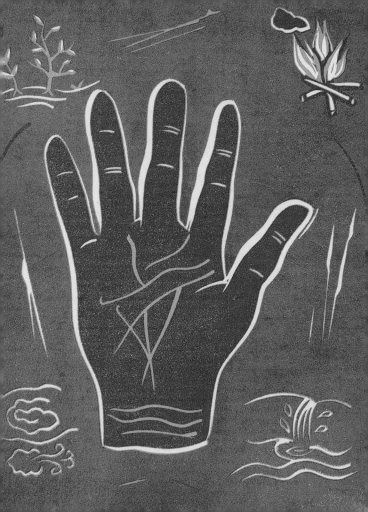

Palms and Lines

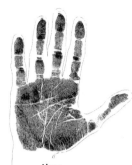

Lines
The lines of the hand can reveal many facets of a person's character.

The lines, and the palm upon which they appear, should be complementary or the inner balance of the subject will be upset.

The square hand implies a precise, methodical, and practical nature, so this type of hand with many lines indicates a sensitive and artistic character, impressionable and, perhaps, with an excess of nervous energy. So it is best for there to be only a few lines on this hand, because if it is covered with lines, the person concerned can become confused easily.

On the conic hand, which indicates sensitivity, we would expect to find many lines, because it is in the nature of the person to be constantly prepared for variety and the stimulus to change. A few lines here suggest the more self-reliant type with a sound constitution and a good balance between nervous energy and physical activity.

It is, therefore, easy to see why the elementary hand has only the few main lines while the psychic hand is covered with a fine tracery of lines. The spatulate hand normally has a reasonable share of lines to reflect the constant activity, while a philosophic hand usually has deeply etched lines emphasizing mental activity.

The more dissimilar a pair of hands, the more changes have been made or imposed on the owner. If the life lines look quite different, family matters or the immediate environment may have been the cause, perhaps in the early years. Health problems may be another reason. If the head lines differ, the subject has had to overcome many problems to achieve his or her aims and may still be doing so. If the heart lines show great differences, then emotional difficulties are the cause.

Weak points

Any interference or fault on any line must obviously detract from its natural strength. A break suggests a lack of continuity, an island is a weakness, and small dots or bars cutting across imply times of serious aggravation.

Occasionally, one or more of the major lines may be missing or so faint as to be virtually nonexistent. The line affected thus becomes a focal point in the nature of the subject.

An absent or weak life line suggests a lack of zest or weak constitution, while a missing heart line reflects poor emotional response or a weakened vascular system.

Comparing Hands

Always remember to check both hands very carefully, for any differences can affect the overall assessment.

SIZES AND SHAPES

Hands are either large or small, but a large person may have relatively small hands, even if they are much larger than those of a small person. Generally, people's hands are relative to their size but occasionally you will find people with hands that are noticeably disproportionate. Large hands cope easily with detail and minor matters. Small hands have little time for such things. All they can see is the finished product and are not concerned when this happens.

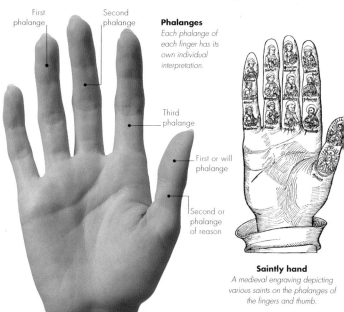

First phalange

Second phalange

Phalanges
Each phalange of each finger has its own individual interpretation.

Third phalange

First or will phalange

Second or phalange of reason

Saintly hand
A medieval engraving depicting various saints on the phalanges of the fingers and thumb.

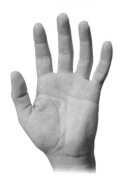

Impulsive

The long palm with short fingers suggests a person who acts on impulse. The smaller the hand the more impulsive the nature.

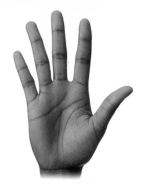

Attention to detail

A long palm with long fingers shows a capacity for detail, but if the palm is short this capacity borders on obsession.

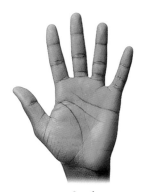

Creative

This long hand together with its spokeshave thumb shows an attraction to the arts.

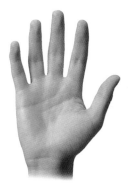

Practical

A square-shaped palm with evenly set fingers denotes a level-headed, practical personality.

Size and Texture

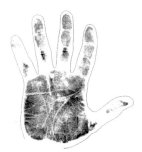

Expressive
A large, expressive hand.
Note the heavy thumb.

The large hand

Large hands belong to people who could be accused of being superficial rather than profound, for they can fritter away their time and talent in endless detail rather than taking in the whole picture. Thus, people with large hands have an analytical mind. Those with large hands with long palms and short fingers are not as impulsive as those with small hands with long palms and short fingers. Memory and attention is only as long as the interest holds them, less if the palms are narrow – in which case the nature may be overfinicky.

Large-handed people with narrow palms are self-centered, subjective, cold, and even ruthless at times. Large hands with short palms and long fingers suggest an obsessive capacity for detail, particularly if there is any knotting at the phalange joints.

A large, broad hand denotes common sense, social ease, and sympathy with the less fortunate. Often, these people are active in welfare or public service, full or part time.

The small hand

Small hands belong to people who envisage the whole without a thought for the detail. They strip an idea to its roots and may be unable to cope with the nuances of a problem.

If the small hands have long palms and short fingers, detail is given some lip service but not for long, for memory is often short-lived unless it concerns something dear to them. People with small hands with long palms and short fingers are impulsive and they rush headlong into projects and schemes, only to find themselves in another scrape from which they need to make their excuses and leave. The memory may be slightly better than with large-handed types, and they may be slightly moody, unless the palms are narrow, in which case they will also be self-centered and petty.

Soft hands

The smaller hand is often soft; physical work is not exactly avoided but it is not pursued either. The person is active mentally, perhaps, but there is almost always a lazy streak.

Hard hands

Large hands are usually firm, implying an active, positive life and straight-forwardness in dealings with others. However, large soft palms suggest a lazy streak and procrastination.

Small Hard Hands

Small hard hands get things done and will connive to get a job finished, no matter what the cost, emotionally, mentally, or even socially.

THE MOUNTS

These are the raised pads found under the base of each finger – Jupiter, Saturn, Apollo, and Mercury – and are collectively called the digital mounts. The third phalange of the thumb forms the mount of Venus, and the large pad on the outer base of the hand is the Luna mount. The small bulge that sometimes appears between them is the Neptune mount. Some palmists ignore the mounts altogether while others scrutinize them for any minute marks. Ideally, the mounts should always be developed, that is, feeling firm and spongy.

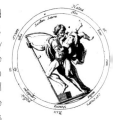

Saturn mount
This should always look developed, for it is the balance of the hand.

Locating the Mounts

○ Jupiter mount – is the first of the digital mounts.

○ The Saturn mount is found immediately under the middle finger.

○ The Apollo mount is found immediately under the third finger.

○ The Mercury mount is rarely found only under the little finger. The third and little fingers often share it, which is perfectly normal.

○ The zone of Mars is in the center of the palm between the digital mounts and the tops of the mounts of Luna and Venus.

○ The Venus mount is really the third phalange of the thumb.

○ The Neptune mount is found at the middle base of the palm.

○ The Pluto mount is a modern idea and is a part of the lower outer third of the mount of the moon.

○ The Luna mount is the padded area halfway down the edge of the palm to the base of the hand.

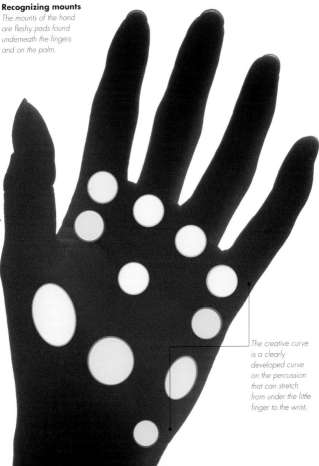

Recognizing mounts

The mounts of the hand are fleshy pads found underneath the fingers and on the palm.

The creative curve is a clearly developed curve on the percussion that can stretch from under the little finger to the wrist.

The Mounts

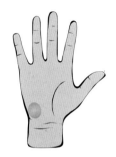

Flat Luna mount
Those with a flat Luna mount lack finesse but can bluff well.

The Jupiter mount

When developed with a centrally placed apex, the subject is actively ambitious, honest, and fond of the good life. If overdeveloped the owner is arrogant, selfish, dictatorial, rude, and direct. A soft or thin mount indicates a lazy streak and a case of the easy way, after making the quick buck every time.

The Saturn mount

If well developed it implies a fatalist who is careful with money and possessions. If overdeveloped, these folk adopt a solitary life and avoid socializing. A flat pad here shows a doubting Thomas, one who just has to spread doom and gloom.

The Apollo mount

This almost always indicates artistic leanings when well developed and once owners put their mind to it they can be very creative. If overdeveloped, the subject has a misplaced sense of self-importance along with a nasty temper and extravagance. A flat mount clearly shows a materialist, selfish and greedy, with little artistic appreciation.

The Mercury mount

When well developed and centrally placed, there will be a flair for business. A well-developed mount suggests people who will bend the rules to suit themselves and may not be honest with themselves or others. He or she may be superstitious. A flat mount implies a poor grasp of the commercial world with weak communication abilities; motivation is weak. This is a follower.

The Venus mount

When well developed there will be
a healthy libido, a warm affectionate
nature, and family life will be important.
If overdeveloped, he or she will be
shameless and oversexed with few
social graces. A flat mount makes these
folk poor company and extremely selfish.

The Neptune mount

When obviously developed this reflects
perceptive and instinctive ways of
understanding what makes people "tick."

The Luna mount

When this is well developed there will
be a vivid imagination along with an
extremely restless nature. There will be
problems keeping to routine. An
overdeveloped mount indicates a lack
of staying power. If flat, it shows a cold
nature with a total lack of imagination.

Mounts and Careers

To find out how the mounts relate to career
success see pages 202–205.

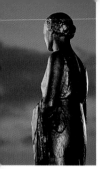

Original ideas
*People with a full-length
creative curve will conceive
and see through innovative
projects from start to finish.*

THE MOUNTS

Other mounts are the zone of Mars in the center of the palm, and the Pluto mount, a modern idea. On the outer edge of some palms a clearly defined curve sometimes seen here is also called a mount, the creative curve. One last mount, the mouse, is formed when the hand is clenched into a fist. If the mounts on both hands are normally soft to the touch, the person's nature might be a bit flat, dull, with a lack of zeal or enthusiasm for life. These types get little out of life but then they don't put a great deal into it either.

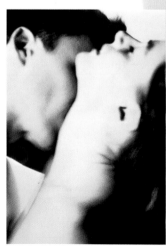

Venus mount
When full and well developed
the overall approach to life is
free of inhibitions. The nature of
the owner is more open and
realistic, often with an open and
healthy libido. If flat and lifeless,
the nature inclines to be
secretive and somewhat closed.

Jupiter mount

When quite full there will be a good approach to social matters; if too full, selfishness and a love of ostentation, vulgar and tasteless in extreme cases. If flat and lifeless, there will be a lazy streak; this is a follower.

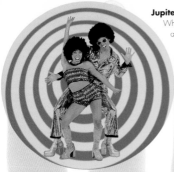

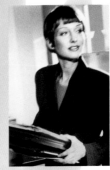

Mercury mount

This usually leans toward its neighbor and when flat suggests a dull personality. The more developed it is, the livelier the owner's overall approach to life.

JUPITER MOUNT

MERCURY MOUNT

VENUS MOUNT

The Mounts

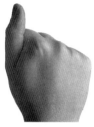

Health mount
A firm bulge here, known as the mouse, indicates current good health.

The zone of Mars

When well developed the owners have good powers of resistance to illness or when things are temporarily going against them. There is a sense of fair play and a strong love of justice. It can also be quite hectic keeping up with such people, for they have so much energy. An overdeveloped zone implies an excess of misplaced zeal and there may be a rebel streak, natural defiance, and hint of cruelty. If underdeveloped these people appear not to have the courage to fight even for what is rightfully theirs and avoid confrontation.

If there is a raised small pad between the first finger and the thumb, then the temper is hard to control and the spirit of competition will be strong. This is the old mount of Mars positive, on the inner edge of the palm, roughly on a par between the head and heart lines – if they reach that far. It shows the owner to have little or no feelings for you or your causes at all. It is a sign of a protestor and a survivor.

The Pluto mount

When well developed there is a practical and theoretical love of occult or secret doctrines. It also seems to be the seat of patriotism. If the padding is very full, the owner has little time for foreigners from anywhere.

The health mount

When the hand is clenched into a fist with the thumb held alongside the index finger, the bulge created on the back of the palm between the thumb and the base of the first finger indicates the current state of our health. When firm to the touch on both hands it shows current good health. When the mount is soft to the touch on the right hand, but firm on the left, our health may be slightly under par, perhaps from tiredness. After a meal and a rest the mount will become firm again and we will feel better.

The creative curve

If the curve is more obvious toward the top of the side of the hand it implies good creative thought; if developed more in the middle, someone who has or who can develop ideas for others to work to. When developed at the base of the side of the hand it suggests the owner can make an idea come alive in practical terms. If the side of the hand is flat or straight the owner is slow to work or appreciate new ideas but may still be clever with his or her hands for this is a feature of the basic square hand.

The Apices

For more information on the significance of the apices on the mounts, see pages 52–53.

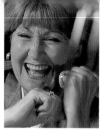

Ambition
The middle horizontal zone of the hand governs our mental nature and the drive to achieve.

THE MODERN APPROACH

In the last 30 years or so a more modern approach has been taken with these traditional areas of the palm, dividing the hand into three vertical areas and three horizontal areas. They each correspond with our conscious and unconscious behavior patterns and the balance we maintain between them. The development or otherwise of the palmar surface shows how well the overall balance is maintained.

Spiritual nature
The top horizontal zone of the hand reflects our spiritual or idealistic nature.

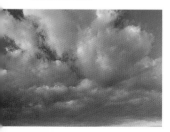

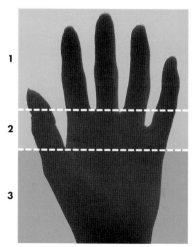

1

2

3

Balance

The lower horizontal zone of the hand represents stability. If this zone is underdeveloped and the middle finger is shorter that the first and third fingers, then the owner lacks common sense and will be involved in reckless pursuits such as gambling.

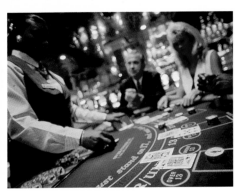

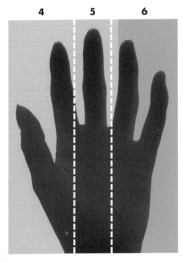

4 5 6

The Zones

The horizontal areas are from the tips of the fingers to where they spring from the top of the hand and from there to a line roughly level to where the top (inner) thumb joins the side of the hand to the wrist. The vertical areas are from the radial side of the hand to between the first and second finger, then from between the middle and third fingers to the ulnar, or outer edge of the hand.

1 The idealist or spiritual nature
2 The mental or ambitious nature
3 The material or basic nature
4 The active or conscious nature
5 The balance of the nature
6 The unconscious or instinctive
   nature

Zones and Areas

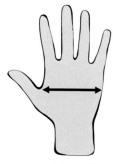

Palm width
*A broad palm implies an open mind;
a narrow palm, limited vision.*

Percussion side

The outer edge of the palm reflects the way we instinctively respond to external stimuli. Thus, a weak-looking or flat ulnar outer edge shows people who find it hard to practice deception. They have difficulty trying to succeed at anything, for they are too open with people.

When well developed the owners can deceive without criminal intent to get the best result for themselves. Bluff is second nature here and you should beware if you oppose them.

Radial side

The radial, or thumb side, of the hand shows how a person is likely to react consciously to external stimuli. A long, well-shaped index finger shows an observant type who takes pride in his or her achievements, and the more the index stands away from the medius, the more sensitive he or she will be.

Middle section

The middle section of the hand is ruled by the Saturn finger and mount. Thus, the development of this area shows how balanced a person's nature will be. As long as the middle finger is long and straight and the Saturn mount well developed, a balanced, stable, and commonsense outlook will prevail.

If this section is not well developed then the owner can be unreliable and out only for what he or she can make with as little effort as possible. If the middle finger is also shorter than the first or third fingers, then he or she may be a gambler, weak-willed, impulsive, and even reckless at times.

Bottom section

The bottom of the hand represents the seat of our energies, and when this area is obviously developed the personality will be more physically inclined, with any mental and emotional pursuits coming a poor second. A wide palm indicates a love of outdoor life or just the freedom such a life brings. A cramped or thin-looking palm implies a selfish nature.

Top section

When the upper area of the palm is well developed and the other zones are fairly balanced, good leadership qualities, perhaps in educational matters, will be present. The subject may well prefer others to lead but takes the role of an adviser, because he or she relishes the idea of being one of the powers behind the throne.

Poor Adaptability

If the first and second fingers are close to each other there is a poor adaptability factor, for this always shows a dislike of anything new.

FULL, EMPTY, OR MEDIUM HANDS

When you see a palm with a vast complexity of lines criss-crossing here, there, and everywhere, it is possible that these may not all be simple influence marks but definite minor lines that can be identified, albeit with some difficulty. However, before dealing with them individually, the overall picture must be assessed first. Trace each of the major lines to establish its path. Note which are influence lines and which are not.

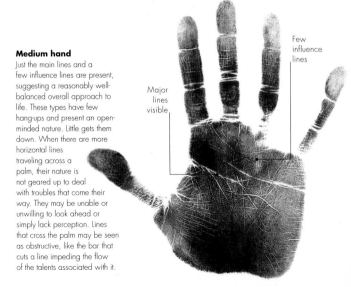

Medium hand

Just the main lines and a few influence lines are present, suggesting a reasonably well-balanced overall approach to life. These types have few hang-ups and present an open-minded nature. Little gets them down. When there are more horizontal lines traveling across a palm, their nature is not geared up to deal with troubles that come their way. They may be unable or unwilling to look ahead or simply lack perception. Lines that cross the palm may be seen as obstructive, like the bar that cuts a line impeding the flow of the talents associated with it.

Major lines visible

Few influence lines

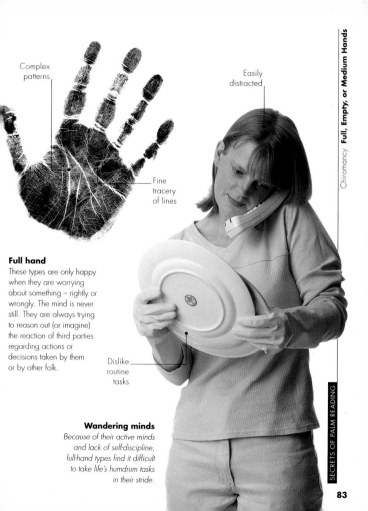

Complex
patterns

Easily
distracted

Fine
tracery
of lines

Full hand

These types are only happy
when they are worrying
about something – rightly or
wrongly. The mind is never
still. They are always trying
to reason out (or imagine)
the reaction of third parties
regarding actions or
decisions taken by them
or by other folk.

Dislike
routine
tasks

Wandering minds

Because of their active minds
and lack of self-discipline,
full-hand types find it difficult
to take life's humdrum tasks
in their stride.

Full and Medium Hands

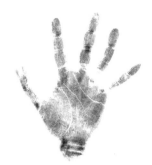

Restless
*A full hand shows a
mind that is never still.*

The full hand

The full hand means exactly that.
It is easy to recognize for there
will be a whole host of lines that
criss-cross all over the palmar surface in
a series of complex patterns. It can be
a palmist's nightmare knowing where to
start to decipher this maze.

This fine tracery of lines is an
indication of someone who worries,
constantly. The mind is never still
because the subject is overemotional
and highly strung. It shows a vivid and
vastly overworked imagination.

These people are often basically
unhappy. They often distrust the motives
of other people and worry about
upsetting those around them and, as a
result, live on a knife's edge. They have
a strangely philosophic approach to life
and many lack confidence.

However, they do not all have
negative qualities – far from it. Many
have brilliant minds and can lead
fascinating lives. While they are also
perceptive, understanding, and really
quite clever, they may just as frequently
lack initiative. These people rarely have
greatness thrust upon them but they
shine when the spotlight picks them up
and places them in the center of things.

They quickly become frustrated with
tasks requiring a lot of attention to
detail, and routine work bores them.
They rarely take kindly to any form of
discipline but they do have a way of
bluffing their way when it comes to
imposing it on other people.

Often found in positions of authority
won early in life because they can
impress with a glib tongue, they do

not often last long because of a lack
of staying power. Many can, therefore,
reach the top but few stay the course,
and when they fail, it takes its toll
inwardly and they suffer with their
nerves, are ill at ease, restless, and
jumpy when the pressures are on.

The medium hand

This type is the mean between the full
and empty hand, for it can be hard to
discern properly and is full of pitfalls for
student palmists. When it is difficult to
be really sure have a check and see
if there are more vertical lines than
horizontal ones on the palm, that is,
if there are more lines traveling up
the palm from the wrist to the fingers.

Vertical lines suggest those who
will always make an effort to seize
every opportunity to improve their
fortunes and better themselves every
chance they get.

Seize the Day

Medium-hand types operate on the basis that,
if you don't try, you won't get anywhere.

THE EMPTY HAND

The empty hand usually has just the three principal lines with a small collection of influence lines or marks dotted about. The empty-handed character has a far steadier and more reliable approach to life and responsibilities. Such folk are relatively free from worries and troubles, and when they do have a problem they keep it to themselves. These people seem not to feel things as deeply as those with the full hands. If they do, it is rare for them to show it.

Empty hand types
They all have a strong tenacity of purpose and once they start something they will finish it – properly. These people refrain from personal touches like kissing or embracing if saying goodbye to or meeting a loved one prior to or after a long absence.

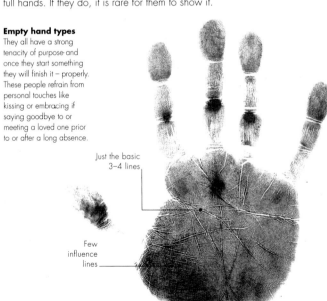

Just the basic 3–4 lines

Few influence lines

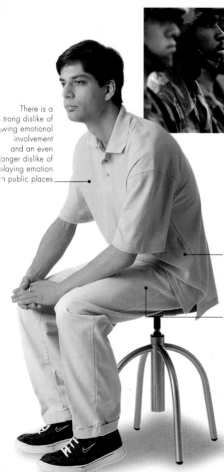

There is a strong dislike of showing emotional involvement and an even stronger dislike of displaying emotion in public places

Regimental
Those with empty hands are extremely suited to all work that involves a disciplined understanding; the armed services suit many of them perfectly. They are conventional and can give or take orders with equal facility.

These people are nearly always straightforward, punctual, and orderly and they love the quiet life

As instructors they excel because they are creative and practical at the same time

Unassuming
They have a very thorough approach and go through life quietly and unobtrusively. Somehow, they simply aren't noticed until it is all over but then it is too late for them – and for you.

The Lines on the Hand

All of us have some but not all of the lines in our hands in some shape or form and as we grow and mature and our character develops, so the lines will reflect these changes. Certain weaknesses will be indicated by faint markings, while strengths are shown by heavily etched lines.

These lines and influence marks are constantly changing as life itself progresses. The palmist has first to establish the shape and style of a hand and only then can begin to decipher their meanings within this context.

Comparing hands

Both hands should be examined. The left hand relates to inherent gifts and talents; the right hand will normally show how well these have been developed.

The reader is invited to experiment as he or she sees fit. As you start to look at hands, make a point of looking at the left hand first and then compare it with the right. No two hands will ever be exactly alike and even the shape may differ. Features such as the texture and

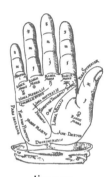

Line map
Early textual figure showing the lines and parts of the hand.

consistency often vary; individual fingers and relative settings do not always exactly match either. As a rule, the right hand is the acknowledged master or dominant because it normally indicates how changes have been absorbed into the personality.

If there are very few differences, the owner has not needed to make changes and thus will exhibit a fairly contented and placid outlook. The more dissimilar the markings, especially an obvious change of shape, the less contented the life. Many significant events will have been experienced, created by the subject or imposed by others.

On a sensitive conic hand one expects to see a fine tracery of lines; on a square hand there may be only a few, which reflects the practical and down-to-earth approach.

When a line divides into an island formation and then reconnects, this obviously suggests a weakness of that line and, by inference, its likely meaning is that enthusiasm for the area of life governed by that line is also weakened, but when the line rejoins the flow of power it regains momentum. Breaks in a line are serious, while dots and crossbars are slightly less so, but they are still a problem, for they break the flow.

Lines that fray or tassellate are often to be seen in elderly hands and show the expected decline of energy.

Clear Lines

The clearer the lines appear the better. Think of them as water pipes. When a break or obstruction occurs, the flow is impeded.

MAJOR AND MINOR LINES

The accepted principal or major lines in the hand are those of head, life, and heart. I personally look to the fate line as a very special case, for it is as important when it is present as it is when it is absent, although it is traditionally classified as a minor line. The maps show the many minor lines as well as the "rings" and the other more important influence marks like, for example, the croix mystique. The meanings of these lines and marks are dealt with in later chapters.

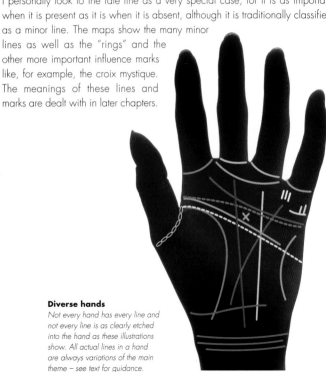

Diverse hands
Not every hand has every line and not every line is as clearly etched into the hand as these illustrations show. All actual lines in a hand are always variations of the main theme – see text for guidance.

Major and Minor Lines

MAJOR LINES	MINOR LINES		
■ Life	■ Sun	■ Ring of Solomon	■ Intuition
■ Heart	■ Mercury	■ Ring of Saturn	■ Via lasciva
■ Head	■ Simian	■ Ring of Apollo	□ Family ring
■ Fate	Sydney	■ Ring of Mercury	Medical stigmata
	■ Rascettes	■ Girdle of Venus	■ Croix mystique
			■ Children and marriage lines

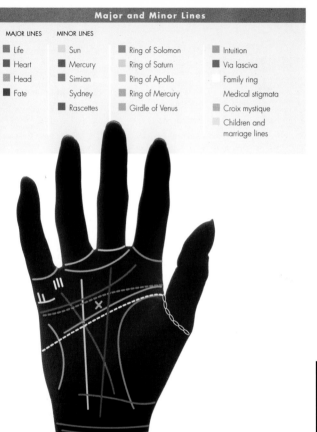

Special Marks and Signs

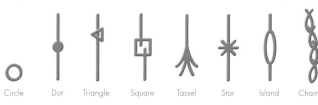

Circle   Dot   Triangle   Square   Tassel   Star   Island   Chain

There is an very wide range of special marks and signs to be found at any point on the palm or fingers. Precisely how many depends on the system used, the school of thought, or the national outlook. In the East there are many marks not recognized in the West but a study of these is worthwhile. Good Eastern palm reading books should list them.

Modern hand analysts may not always use the 14 listed here and not all of these will be found on any one hand. It is quite possible none of these will appear but at least 4 or 5 are likely to be seen in any one pair of hands.

These special marks are, in alphabetical order, the bar, chain, circle, cross, dot, grille, island, square, star, tassel, triangle, trident, and horizontal or vertical line.

Meanings

They may be on their own, or be part of a line, perhaps with other marks formed accidentally by a junction of major or minor lines. Generally, the circle, square, star, triangle, trident, and vertical line are said to be beneficial and are often found on the hand.

All of the other marks – the bar, chain, cross, dot, grille, island, and tassel – are considered detrimental but dependent on where they are found.

Study them carefully, for they are a bit like the minor aspects you find in astrology and are often the answer to a detail of personality for which there may be no immediate or obvious answer.

In some cases they may refer to an incident from the past that the subject has chosen to remember because of the effect it had at the time.

Cross and
Grille

Vertical and
horizontal Lines

Trident
and Bar

They may be a warning sign for
something that may come to pass at
a later date.

For example, wherever the square
is seen it is always favorable and
recognized as a sign of preservation.
If the life line looks strong after passing
by one it could refer to a short period in
the hospital. However, a star near the
end of the life line denotes a shock and
should be seen as a warning sign.

The circle on a line is easy to
mistake for an island or a badly
formed square or triangle and must
be examined carefully. The trident is
a feature of Indian palm reading.

The Unforeseen

For further information on the significance of
the special marks and the unforeseen see
pages 214–217.

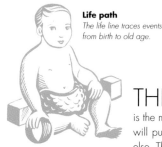

Life path
The life line traces events from birth to old age.

THE LIFE LINE

When this line is the most heavily emphasized then the subject will put the physical above almost everything else. This type of line is more likely to be found on the hands of those folk who prefer the great outdoors and thrive when involved in physical activities. However, like any of the other lines, it must never be read in isolation but always be assessed in conjunction with them and other features in a hand if you are to make a satisfactory analysis of the person whose hands are under review.

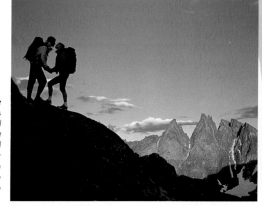

The great outdoors
A heavily etched life line will reflect a strongly physical attitude to life, whether the subject is an athlete or someone who prefers to work outdoors.

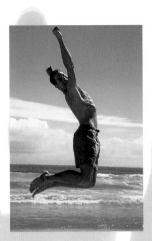

Zest for living

An uninterrupted, strongly etched line indicates enthusiasm and a sparkling nature. Almost always a person of this type has a zest for living.

The life line can start almost anywhere on the radial side of the hand usually on the Jupiter or Mars mount or between them. It may begin within the skin pattern at the extreme radial edge of the palm or quite a way inside it

It often starts as a chained or islanded affair but it should be a very clearly etched single path that sweeps firmly out into the palm, encircling the mount of Venus, and ending somewhere near the base of the hand

Reading the Life Line

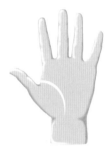

Outdoor types
A strongly etched life line suggests that the owner enjoys physical life.

The life line is the most important gauge of our constitution and vitality and it should always look strong and healthy. The more interruptions on the line the less its power to operate as it should.

Sometimes the line appears to constrict the ball of the thumb and tuck in under the mount of Venus. It can sweep outward to end anywhere on the Luna mount or be the division between the two bottom mounts. In a few cases it can travel on to the lower outer edge of the palm. It can fork into several branches, fade away, fray, or tassellate.

Life line beginnings

When it starts as a single line within the skin pattern at the edge of the palm the nature is open and self-reliant, but when it is chained, then the owner will be too reliant on others. An open-ended island formation suggests an element of mystery surrounding birth, adoption, or illegitimacy or, perhaps, difficulty with the physical birth.

When, at the start, it is tied with the head line, the longer they stay together, the more cautious their owner in relationships with others. These folk will be hypersensitive, full of self-doubt, and difficult to understand; they tend to achieve very little. There can be a hint of national pride or a love of family tradition, the right way of getting things done – convention is important to them.

As the life line moves away from the head line little influence lines may be seen between them. When there are many of them, the nature is not very positive and the owners will look to others for leadership, because they lack any real decisiveness themselves.

A line that begins high up on the mount of Jupiter denotes a healthy, driving, ambitious nature. These people will be confident and feel they are infallible. When things go wrong, they must find someone else to blame rather than admit they were wrong. The lower down the beginning of this line, the less this tendency. The nature will be open, friendly, and natural.

A life line that originates from the mount of Mars and clings tightly around the ball of the thumb creates a sensitive, touchy soul, ready to kick in a self-defense mechanism at the slightest sign of trouble. A line rising on the Mars mount suggests the subject is a follower who rarely moves without checking every step of the way and even then hesitates. A line touching or passing through the line from inside the life line, shows an interfering family member or close friend.

Timing Events

For information on timing events using the life line, see pages 190–97.

THE LIFE LINE

Traditionally, it has always been thought that a short line implies a short life and a long line implies a long life. This is quite wrong, for there are many folk who have just a token marking or perhaps have no life line at all on either hand. While it is true that they are not very strong physically and may have a weaker than average constitution, such people can and do live to a ripe old age.

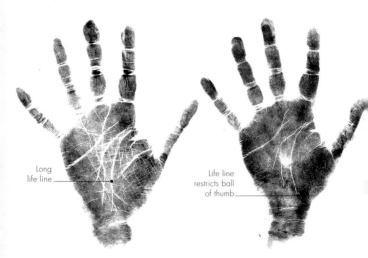

Long life line

Life line restricts ball of thumb

Long life line

A long life line usually suggests someone who prefers to work more with physical things than abstract matters.

Line restricts ball of thumb

In cases where the life line restricts the ball of the thumb there is little enthusiasm for life and there may be a restricted overall outlook.

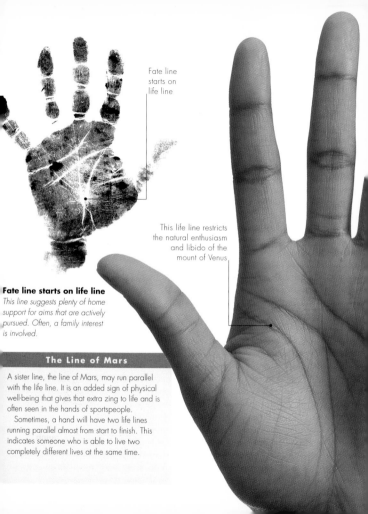

Fate line
starts on
life line

This life line restricts
the natural enthusiasm
and libido of the
mount of Venus

Fate line starts on life line
*This line suggests plenty of home
support for aims that are actively
pursued. Often, a family interest
is involved.*

The Line of Mars

A sister line, the line of Mars, may run parallel
with the life line. It is an added sign of physical
well-being that gives that extra zing to life and is
often seen in the hands of sportspeople.

Sometimes, a hand will have two life lines
running parallel almost from start to finish. This
indicates someone who is able to live two
completely different lives at the same time.

Reading the Life Line

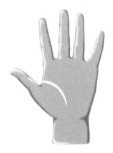

Short life line
A short life line does not signify a short life.

Influence marks that stem from the palmar area, outside the life line, indicate from where or from whom problems originate: if from Jupiter, a career matter perhaps; if from Saturn, personal discipline; or if from the Apollo finger or mount, artistic or creative matters. If a line comes from the Mercury finger or mount it relates to commercial matters.

When the life line in the right hand sweeps out into the palmar surface with little or no ties between it and the head line, the owner will make continuous conscious efforts to better his or her life.

If the left-hand line seems to restrict the ball of the thumb but the right-hand line is noticeably different and sweeps right out into the palm, there will be many attempts to better the life. These subjects consider their early years were disadvantageous and difficult to cope with and that this held them back. They will have faced up to overbearing parents, risen above scholastic or environmental dissatisfaction, and recognized health weaknesses with a sensible and responsible regimen.

The reverse of this, when the left-hand line sweeps out into the palm but the right-hand line stays close to the mount of Venus, indicates depleted circumstances that have taken their toll. The owner has made the best of things but, while aware of these problems, was unable or unwilling to do anything about them and has let things slide.

Influence lines rising up from the life line show efforts made to improve the standard of living and, if long enough, they should indicate in which direction the owner is or was aiming.

Breaks in the line

Once halfway down the hand the line may break up to end in a number of different ways but, when there is little change in its appearance, the owners will be content and in control of their affairs. Little upsets them, and they can bend with the wind quite well. When there are changes, it will be at about middle age. At this time most ambitions have been or are nearly achieved.

At this point the line might look strong, but a little lower down it might begin to break up, showing signs of stress. The owner has taken on too much; the line is giving an early warning and they should take steps to ease matters, or else.

Life Line and Travel

If the line curves in under the ball of the thumb there is a dislike of travel or being away. This person likes to return home, the one place he or she feels secure. A life line that sweeps out and ends on the Luna mount indicates a love of travel and fresh experiences. It is the clearest mark of travel in a hand, and stressed if in both hands. A forked end indicates restlessness; and the owner will be involved in activities that will reflect this

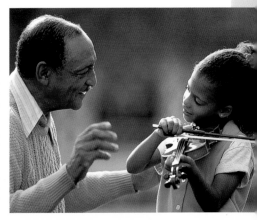

Imagination

When a head line is long and strong, the imaginative side of the subject's nature will be quite active, and he or she will be easily sidetracked.

THE HEAD LINE
I have always considered the head line to be the most important on a hand, for it shows the way you think and reason, perceive and believe, and how you then apply the information after digesting all the facts. We all think and act in our own fashion. As a result, we assume a lifestyle based on this thinking. Because of all the wide-ranging differences it is reasonable to expect the head line to start from a variety of places and take its own path on the surface of the hand.

Talent
The head line on the right hand will show the development of talents suggested by the head line on the left hand. Any perceptible differences show what changes have been made – or are still being made. The greater these differences, the more changes the character will experience.

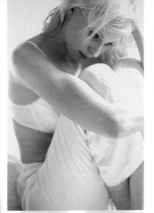

Uncertainty

When the head line begins just inside the life line, either just touching it or slightly away from it, this suggests uncertainty or a lack of confidence.

The ideal head line begins very near the life line on the radial side of the hand and sweeps out into the palmar surface

✕

It will start to bow slightly and slope gently down to end on the top of the Luna mount

✕

The ideal ending is somewhere under the little finger along the outer edge of the hand. More often than not, it may be a little or a long way short of it

Reading the Head Line

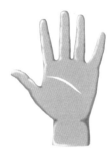

Line of reason
The head line governs the way in which we use our reasoning abilities.

The head line may start from anywhere on the Jupiter mount, which indicates pride in achievement. It sometimes starts a short distance away from the life line. The farther away from the life line, the more rash and impulsive the nature, especially if found on a conic hand. It may take a straight path across the middle of the hand or slope slightly. Occasionally, it will dip steeply to end on the Luna mount. It may end suddenly, fork once or twice, tassellate or fray, or just fade out.

Comparing hands

When you compare the head lines on both hands, one will seem to be more strongly drawn than the other. If the weaker line is on the right hand, the thinking will be negative, vacillating, and submissive. When the weaker line is on the left hand, the reasoning powers will be positive and well ordered. The owner will have used his or her initiative to break free from possible early restrictions.

When both lines are of equal intensity with similar origins and follow the same paths, the owner will experience few changes.

Length

A short line indicates a practical nature, less flexible than average. The subject may achieve fame or infamy for specialist abilities. A short line that ends under the middle finger is not usually seen on the conic hand but is more likely to be found on a square hand. It shows a good, practical level of concentration. It also indicates concern with mundane matters and a flair for routine. A long head line implies cluttered thinking but with a more flexible approach. These people are very imaginative.

The long head line that extends to the outer edge of the palm, virtually cutting a hand in two, is called a Sydney line. It shows excellent mental control, an inflexible nature, and a very strong selfish streak.

Occasionally, you may see hands that bear a head line with an irregular appearance. It starts strongly, fades away, then comes back again. This shows a struggle to keep one's head above water, an inability to cope. Influence lines or other marks at this point in the head line should show the cause. The higher the head line starts on the mount of Jupiter, the more honorable the character.

Double Head Line

Occasionally, a double head line is seen and indicates an ability to exist or work in completely different spheres of activity at the same time.

THE HEAD LINE

Like all lines, the head line should be clear of any influence marks except for those vertical lines that are expected to cross. There must be no dots, bars, islands, chaining, furring, or fraying. The clearer the line, the clearer the thought processes. The more the line slopes the more imagination is present and used.

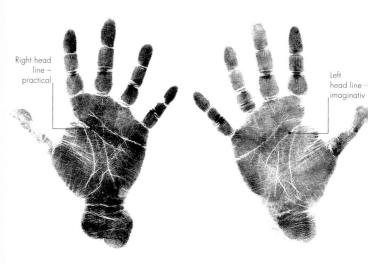

Right head line – practical

Left head line – imaginative

Different head lines

These two prints are from a hairdresser's palms. The left-hand line shows an imaginative nature but is not very practical. The right-hand line turns up very slightly which suggests that the owner realized her mental or creative approach could

be turned to the more practical side of things. Thus, the woman decided to work for herself as a hairdresser. Whenever the head line lifts upward, no matter how slightly, there is an ability to earn money with the owner's personal talents – for good or ill.

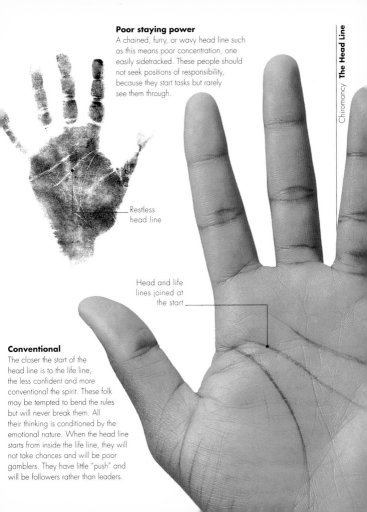

Poor staying power

A chained, furry, or wavy head line such as this means poor concentration, one easily sidetracked. These people should not seek positions of responsibility, because they start tasks but rarely see them through.

Restless head line

Head and life lines joined at the start

Conventional

The closer the start of the head line is to the life line, the less confident and more conventional the spirit. These folk may be tempted to bend the rules but will never break them. All their thinking is conditioned by the emotional nature. When the head line starts from inside the life line, they will not take chances and will be poor gamblers. They have little "push" and will be followers rather than leaders.

Reading the Head Line

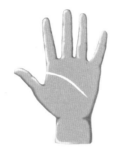

Imaginative
A head line sweeping into the Luna mount reveals an imaginative mind.

People with a heavily etched line love flattery, and the deeper the line, the more egotistic the nature. A wide gap between the start of the head and life lines shows an impulsive nature; while they are ambitious and capable of carrying through plans, they antagonize people with their lack of tact.

The longer and more even the rectangular space between the head and heart lines the more common sense prevails. The wider the space, the more practicality rules, while the narrower the space the more emotional the character.

The head line and the mounts

If the head line rises up to the mount of Mercury, the nature is cold; emotion is cut out of relationships. This is much the same as when the line remains high above the central part of the hand – again, all feeling and warmth is taken out of personal relationships. On both hands, this means that all emotional considerations will be subjected to the demands of the mind.

When the head line sweeps down the palm deep into the Luna mount there will be an active imagination but the lower the line reaches, the less positive the mental faculties. If the line fades at the end, this trait will be emphasized.

Islands, forks, and influence lines

An island on any part of the head line suggests a weakening of the power of the whole line. If the head line forks at the end it indicates contrasting elements in the life of the owner, showing an active mentality that is well suited to research work. If the fork is toward the end of a line there is an ability to pursue two different careers at the same time.

Influence lines rising from the head line always refer to efforts made by the subject to improve his or her standing. Lines that fall away suggest poor decision-making with attendant losses.

When the head line fades toward its end it is merely reflecting weakness that comes with age. Those who have this line should be prepared to slow down and relinquish responsibilities as gracefully as they can. The hand is advising that their natural energies will wane as they age and they must learn to live with this. When the head line looks stronger than the life line, the intellectual side will predominate.

Writer's Hook

A small or shorter fork at the end of a forked head line that turns slightly upward is fancifully called the "writer's hook" but is not limited to writing and covers any other creative pursuit. If one of the lines reaches the percussion the owner is liable to receive international recognition (fame or infamy) depending on the nature of the endeavors.

Emotional

A deeply grooved line of heart suggests that the subject has strong emotional feelings.

THE HEART LINE

The line of heart governs our emotional responses and the way that they shape our character and personality. It also indicates the level of vascular health and in certain circumstances can also show hearing and sight defects. The more curved the heart line appears the more emotionally responsive the subject; the straighter the line, the less flexible the nature. A lightly marked heart line line may indicate a highly sensitive, slightly shy type.

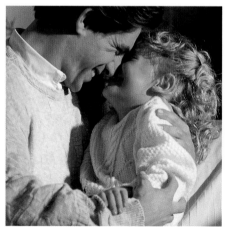

Low-set heart line

People with low-set heart lines always show depth of feeling in their dealings with everybody, especially the younger folk. They are far more in touch with their emotions and much more responsive than those in the older generations.

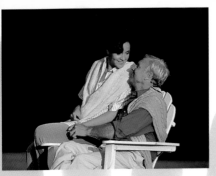

Affectionate side

Look to the heart line to show the depth of understanding and the affectionate side of our nature. The physical nature of love and our emotions are shown by the depth that the heart line sinks into the palm. The higher and straighter the line in the palm, the less physically expressive the nature.

A high start on the Jupiter mount suggests a supporting role in a relationship

The line should be clear and positive throughout, but this is rarely the case. There are often islands or chain formations

A short line that does not reach the percussion suggests dedication to a cause or an ideal

Reading the Heart Line

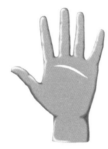

Short heart line
*A short, straight high-set heart line
may indicate a cold nature.*

There are two distinctive schools of thought concerning this particular line. It has always been accepted that the line starts on the radial side of the hand where the other two main lines have their beginnings.

Because emotions are instinctive there are those who argue that the heart line must start on the percussion and travel to the radial side of the hand. In turn, this has produced a small minority of people who claim that the line cannot have a beginning or an end because of what it represents.

Further, as this line often begins with a fork and the other two generally end in one, the issue has produced some lively discussions.

The heart line may begin on or just under the mount of Jupiter, between the first and second fingers, or in the skin pattern at the radial edge of the hand just above the head line. It can also start on the mount of Saturn with a fork on the mount under the first finger.

If the heart line starts high up and remains there, this suggests an idealist. When the line forks with one branch from the radial edge and the other from the mount of Jupiter it indicates emotional adaptability. Often, when this line does fork a branch stems from the Saturn mount, with the other from the radial edge, one line etched a little more strongly than the other.

If the stronger branch originates from the side of the hand, the nature will be proud and honest. The other way around shows an open and practical outlook and is often seen on the hands of carers.

Length and density

It may be thick or thin, long or short, chained or islanded and should always be free of influence marks except for those that cross it as a matter of course.

A deeply marked line suggests emotional pressure with attendant health troubles – worry, stress, and strain. But this line can often seem darker than the other two main lines and what these illnesses are ought to be confirmed elsewhere in the hand.

A short, straight, high-set heart line implies a cold emotional outlook. This will be emphasized with a narrow palm. A low-set heart line shows a passionate character and if the head line is also set low there will be possessiveness.

The Perfect Heart Line

The perfect line commences under the first finger and pursues a gently curving path all the way to the percussion. This indicates a healthy and reasonably well-balanced nature emotionally. The lower the line dips into the palm the more physical that nature will be expressed. The higher heart line implies a more mental approach.

THE HEART LINE

Quite often the heart line is the darkest or most heavily etched line in the hand, suggesting that subjects obey their emotional instincts despite what the mind or common sense tells them to do. When this happens there are often many little influence lines that drop away into the palm toward the head line. The higher the heart line stays along the top of the palm, the less this will be so.

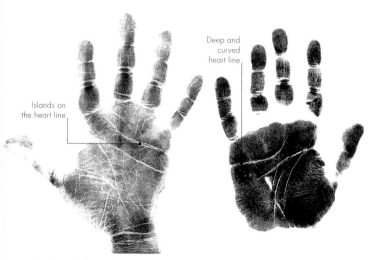

Deep and curved heart line

Islands on the heart line

Islands in the heart line

An island in the heart line just below the middle finger can suggest hearing problems, while one under the third finger may reflect sight troubles. If found on both hands these troubles may be emphasized.

Deep and curved heart line

The deeper the heart line curves or reaches into the palm, the more depth of feeling there will be. The straighter and higher the line, the more matter of fact the emotional approach.

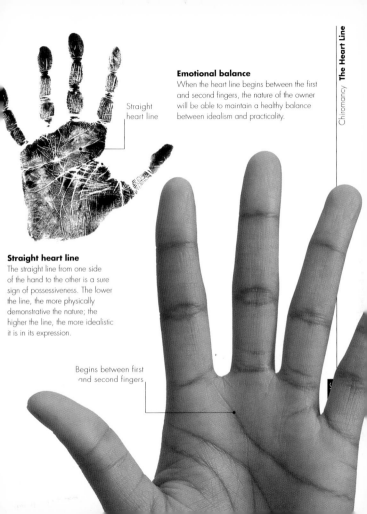

Straight
heart line

Emotional balance
When the heart line begins between the first
and second fingers, the nature of the owner
will be able to maintain a healthy balance
between idealism and practicality.

Straight heart line
The straight line from one side
of the hand to the other is a sure
sign of possessiveness. The lower
the line, the more physically
demonstrative the nature; the
higher the line, the more idealistic
it is in its expression.

Begins between first
and second fingers

Reading the Heart Line

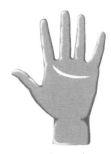

Responsive
If the line curves or dips sharply into the palm, the nature is much warmer.

When the heart line ends on the outer edge under the mount of Mercury, more on the mount of Mars, the emotional nature will be selfish, cold, and unforgiving.

If all three of the main lines are connected at the start it warns of a traumatic shock to the system – the kind of incident never forgotten and from which the subject may never recover.

A faint heart line suggests a less passionate outlook, people who go through many affairs more for physical rather than emotional satisfaction.

They are also quite direct, with their feet on the ground, and are self-protective. Despite this outlook, they are relatively open and friendly until trouble rears its head, then it's every man for himself – and they are first in line.

A heart line with a low start, between the thumb and index finger, shows a possessive nature, emphasized the farther it stretches across the hand. These folk cannot abide criticism of those whom they trust and it is very difficult to persuade them otherwise.

People with straight heart lines are not so warm and easy to get along with; they are inhibited and not easily persuaded. The curved line shows a far more demonstrative nature – much warmer, more open and friendly.

Left and right hand

Significant changes between heart lines in a pair of hands are often noted. The deeper etched line in the left hand with a more practical line on the right shows the subject to have been hurt in an earlier relationship. The reverse of this indicates a sympathetic partner who has drawn the subject out of his or her shell. If there is little difference, this shows someone with a contented nature.

Influence lines

A restless outlook is shown by tiny influence lines that fall away from the line as it starts. This can be carried to extremes in that the subject might vary travel arrangements for the sake of change. There will be few really close friends, but a wide and varied circle of acquaintances. Knowledge tends to be somewhat superficial; they are Jacks or Jills of all trades who know a little about many widely differing subjects and take things as they come.

Health and the Heart Line

Dental, hearing, and sight defects can be found on this line. A little island in the line under the Saturn finger suggests hearing problems and there may be a fear of heights.

An island on the line under the Apollo finger is associated with eye or sight defects. Three or four vertical lines just above the heart line under the Mercury finger may indicate dental troubles.

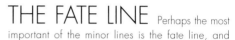

Family values

A child with no fate line on either hand requires firm guidance from his or her parents.

THE FATE LINE

Perhaps the most important of the minor lines is the fate line, and in practice I treat this as the fourth major line, for it is essential to observe whether it is missing from the hand, just as much as to examine it when it is there. Either way, present or not, give this line as much attention as you can reasonably spare. Its influence can be equally as strong when it is not present as when it is there.

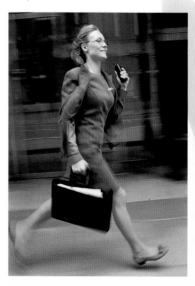

Full fate line

The fate line indicates an awareness of responsibilities and the owner does his or her best to maintain their role, which also helps them to establish their position in society. People with a full fate line are upright, honest, and straightforward and understand their role in society. Often they work where precision is essential. It is rare to find a full-length fate line in both hands but when it is present the owner has an intuitive awareness of his or her environment. Also, it imposes limitations because it governs the desires and ambitions of the subject and these may be beyond his abilities.

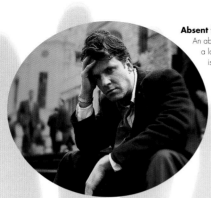

Absent fate line
An absent line always shows a lack of direction. The subject is unsure and unsettled with little personal pride in himself or his appearance.

The fate line starts at the wrist and goes directly to the base of the middle finger. A variation of this path is not a fate line in the real sense but one of several associated lines: the awareness, destiny, environment or milieu, and direction or duty lines

Reading the Fate Line

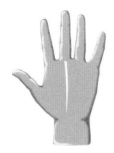

Present or absent?
*The fate line is significant
whether it is present or not.*

The fate line is important, for it is heavily involved in our nature and general approach to life. None of the other major lines have this special quality. If there is no line of head, heart, and life it has no special significance.

When there is no fate line on either hand of a young child, he or she should be given a fairly strict upbringing and taught the essentials of life as early as possible. The difference between right and wrong needs to be understood early on to ensure that the child will not fritter his or her life away.

The beginning of the fate line

The true fate line starts among the rascettes or inside the life line from the mount of Venus which, strictly speaking, makes it a duty line. For as long as it is inside the life line, the owner is subject to the family wishes. When you see this, examine the fate line as it leaves the life line. If it looks stronger the youngster followed the family wishes and is making the most of his or her new career. However, if the fate line weakens or fades out, an effort may have been made but was later abandoned. Sometimes a new line starts as this one ends – a strong line shows confidence and promise for the new venture.

The fate line that begins from the life line implies restriction in the early years. The youngster will have had to work hard to achieve what he or she has. The higher the line starts, the later in life the owner will follow a chosen direction.

The fate line can also start from anywhere on the Luna mount. A long clear line to the base of the middle finger indicates independence and a very determined nature. It is likely that the career depends on public approbation for success – singing, dancing, acting, or possibly politics.

A forked beginning to a fate line suggests two distinct sides to the subject's ambitions. If a branch from the Venus mount meets with a line from the Luna mount the subject is aware of what he or she is supposed to do regarding family wishes. The stronger of the two forks will show who wins in the end.

The milieu line

A short line sometimes appears between the life and fate line but stops before the head line. This is the milieu line and it is a sign of trouble. It prevents the owner from achieving the aim of the moment through ill-health, insufficient money, or people who interfere without just cause. When the line stops, so do the problems.

Timing Events

For information on using the fate line to time events, see page 196.

THE FATE LINE

It is imperative not to underestimate the importance of the fate line, whether it is there or not. When it is absent, there is no real sense of direction. When it is there – and, as a rule, there is almost always some semblance of the line present, no matter how long or short it is – the owner will have some sort of aim in life. This line maintains an overall balanced approach. The stronger it is, the more some semblance of self-control will be present. When only lightly etched, the nature can be vacillating.

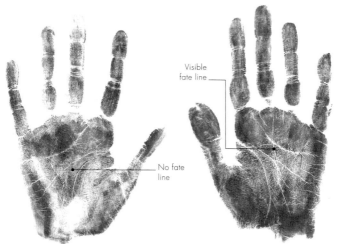

Visible fate line

No fate line

Comparing right and left

If a fate line is found only on the right hand this shows subjects with the ability always to try to better themselves, and their initiative is usually quite strong.

When in the left hand only it shows dreams and aspirations but little ability to pursue them. The above examples show an excellent fate line in the right hand, with nothing in the left.

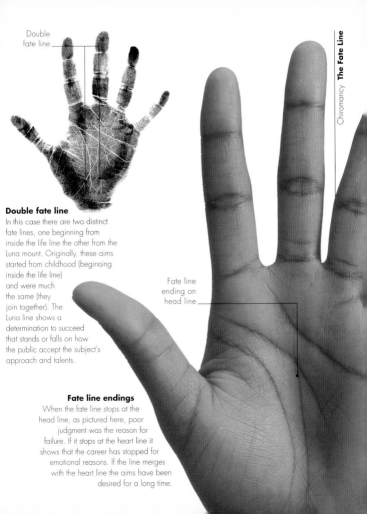

Double
fate line

Double fate line

In this case there are two distinct
fate lines, one beginning from
inside the life line the other from the
Luna mount. Originally, these aims
started from childhood (beginning
inside the life line)
and were much
the same (they
join together). The
Luna line shows a
determination to succeed
that stands or falls on how
the public accept the subject's
approach and talents.

Fate line
ending on
head line

Fate line endings

When the fate line stops at the
head line, as pictured here, poor
judgment was the reason for
failure. If it stops at the heart line it
shows that the career has stopped for
emotional reasons. If the line merges
with the heart line the aims have been
desired for a long time.

Reading the Fate Line

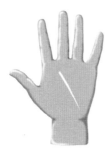

Variation
This shorter variation of the fate line begins from the Luna mount.

The clearer the fate line, the more success is likely, although this does not necessarily mean fame and fortune. The line shows how much real, inner satisfaction the subject will enjoy through his or her efforts. Money and fame as a result is an added bonus.

When the line starts quite faint and then strengthens, the owner will have experienced a poor start before everything took off. When the fate line starts from the Luna mount and travels to the Jupiter finger there is always good personal motivation.

Forks and branches

When the line breaks into many little branches at the end, the owner will diversify so much that nothing will be satisfactorily achieved. Sometimes when the fate line forks, one branch goes to the Jupiter mount and the other to Saturn. Where the fork starts is important: at the head line, a business matter perhaps; while at the heart line, it shows an emotional change of heart.

Traditionally, a trident fork at the end of a line is very lucky but only if the line branches after passing the heart line. The fate line from the wrist to middle finger suggests the owner is a fatalist. Everything is put down to a sense of duty and obligation. Life is spent in a rut with no attempt to get out of it.

Fulfilling ambitions

Lines that fade and return show weak and strong periods. The fate line that starts between the head and the heart lines implies a long-felt ambition that the owner has finally been able to pursue actively. If it starts from the heart line the subject has been fascinated by the interest first as a hobby and has now turned it into a successful career. Look to the palmar skin pattern for verification. Between the Jupiter and Saturn fingers a clearly defined loop will be seen to enter the palm, the loop of serious intent, which shows that such a long-felt desire may one day become a reality.

If it begins between the heart line and the base of the fingers the exact location of its beginning will be crucial: on the mount of Jupiter, a career move; on Saturn, a long-desired position of responsibility; on the Apollo mount, it will be in one of the creative arts; and on the Mercury mount, something to do with communications, which in turn depends on the hand shape.

Time and the Fate Line

Provided you accept that the line of fate proper begins at the wrist and ends at the base of the first finger, a sense of time can be safely assumed. It is generally acknowledged that where the fate line crosses the head line is, on average, the 35th year and where it crosses the heart line is about the 50th year.

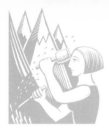

Concentration

Those with a Simian line channel their energy into a furious, concentrated onslaught on the task at hand.

THE SIMIAN AND SYDNEY LINES

The Simian line is created when the head line fuses with the heart line and produces one line across the top of the palm. If this has always been the case, the line is fairly straightforward looking. But sometimes the two lines have started separately and have since grown together and formed this one line, in which case it may look scrappy and incomplete. The Sydney line occurs when the head line is sometimes seen to sweep over the palmar surface in one straight line as if cutting it in two.

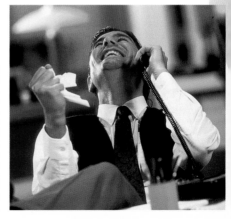

High achievers

People with a Simian line are obsessives: they must succeed, they have to win and must never be diverted from their ambitions. To achieve is all they know – not necessarily a large and grandiose project, but the aim of the moment. If a letter has to be written it has to be done now. It could be the shopping or a journey – no matter what the aim, it takes on an exaggerated importance.

Control freaks

Those with a Sydney line possess great mental control and will not let emotions sway them when it comes to achieving an ambition. If this line appears in both hands the owner will be extremely ruthless and stop at nothing to pursue his or her aims.

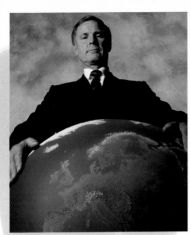

Usual course of heart line

Sydney line – when the head line cuts the palm in two

The Simian line. When the two major influences of mind and emotion are fused into one line it is only natural to expect an increased intensity of purpose – for better or for worse

Usual course of head line

The Simian and Sydney Lines

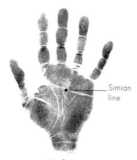

Simian line

Perfect
This hand print shows a perfect Simian line.

The Simian line

Even normally articulate and quite intelligent people who have this line can become power-mad, when the mood takes them. They become so caught up with the need to achieve their aims that nothing, and no one, gets in their way; they are unable to direct their talents as they should.

There is always a sense of purpose; they seem different; you feel their ability to control, to be always right and not to make mistakes. They must always have the facts, never probabilities. Social niceties will be dispensed with and they become efficient machines; personal popularity is the last thing on their minds.

When the Simian line lies deep into the palm the emotional side of the nature is badly controlled, but when it is set higher in the hand the intellectual side is more dominant.

When this line is fairly thick at its commencement, the personality is quite cold and calculating. If it is more strongly etched toward the outer edge of the hand, the emotions are instinctive. One straight, thick line right across the hands shows a selfish and materialistic nature.

A thinner or more lightly etched line implies a highly sensitive inner nature coupled with natural intuition. Reactions are fast but always with that selfish side of their natures in evidence. These folk are often very restless and they cannot stay still for long.

The Sydney line

This indicates people who can cut all emotion from their lives and operate in a cold, precise manner for as long as it takes to achieve the current aim.

If in both hands, the mental control exercised is formidable; these are people quite prepared to sacrifice everything to win. In the left hand only, it shows people who cannot accept criticism or rejection. However, they have long memories – they never forget or forgive any slight, no matter how unintentional it may have been.

In the right hand only it marks selfishness; people who take great pride in their achievements and who will not acknowledge help. But there is still great mental control over all the emotional life and reactions.

No Half Measures

Those with a Simian line love or hate with equal intensity. It does not pay to oppose them unless you are sure of your facts.

THE MERCURY LINE

The Mercury line has had many names and may still be called the health line or Hepatica, the liver line, the line of stomach, and, of late, the business line. Students have been known to confuse it with the line of intuition. When found in the hand, no matter how badly or well formed it may be, much of its path lies on the unconscious or passive side and suggests an inner awareness of health in a general sense.

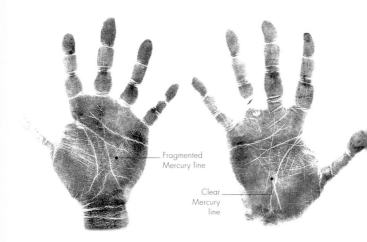

Fragmented Mercury line

Clear Mercury line

Badly formed Mercury line
This hand shows a badly formed Mercury line. The actual formation of the line is not significant because the owners of any type of Mercury line will be conscious of their health, sometimes even to the point of hypochondria.

Well-formed Mercury line
When the Mercury line begins from the life line itself there is almost always a concern with diet and health. The subjects will dislike taking pills, tinctures, or any other form of relief. They would rather suffer a headache than relieve it.

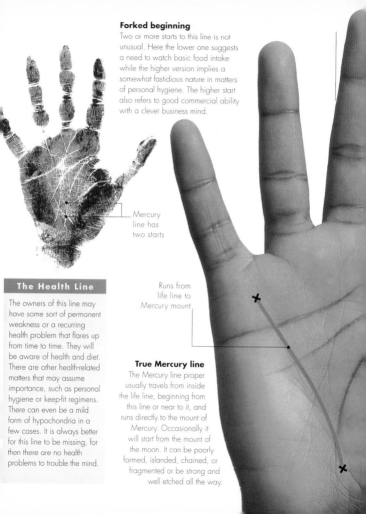

Forked beginning

Two or more starts to this line is not unusual. Here the lower one suggests a need to watch basic food intake while the higher version implies a somewhat fastidious nature in matters of personal hygiene. The higher start also refers to good commercial ability with a clever business mind.

Mercury line has two starts

Runs from life line to Mercury mount

The Health Line

The owners of this line may have some sort of permanent weakness or a recurring health problem that flares up from time to time. They will be aware of health and diet. There are other health-related matters that may assume importance, such as personal hygiene or keep-fit regimens. There can even be a mild form of hypochondria in a few cases. It is always better for this line to be missing, for then there are no health problems to trouble the mind.

True Mercury line

The Mercury line proper usually travels from inside the life line, beginning from this line or near to it, and runs directly to the mount of Mercury. Occasionally it will start from the mount of the moon. It can be poorly formed, islanded, chained, or fragmented or be strong and well etched all the way.

The Mercury Line

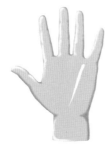

Long and straight
A long, straight Mercury line may suggest self-delusion or inhibitions.

When the Mercury line starts from the mount of Venus, inside the life line, it implies that the subject is a born worrier. There may be a weakness of the digestive system and a tendency either to avoid or take supplementary remedies and vitamins regularly.

When the allergy line (see page 134) is also found in the hand, then allergies, real or imagined, will be a feature. In many cases, you name the ailment, they have had it. Just talking about health and suffering is enough for these people.

The business line

When the Mercury line begins in the central zone of Mars, away from and not touching the life line, aversions to taking pills and remedies are not so obvious. When this happens the line should now be regarded as the business line. Big business, industry, and commerce of all kinds attract, and the type of hand upon which the line is found will indicate the main interest.

These people seem to have a natural flair for finance. Often, this is the sign of the good salesperson, someone who is able to interpret trends and know exactly how and when to seize the opportunity to make money.

When the Mercury line crosses the head line, if it is long enough, any influence lines seen passing between them often indicate an interest in the occult. The rest of the hand will show how this is to be interpreted. Should the line break up as it passes through the head line, a number of varying interests will concern the owner. A love of ritual and formal procedure may be present.

When this line has a number of small segments passing the head line on the Luna mount, the imagination knows no bounds. If the head line is forked and the Mercury line passes over both branches, the person will be hypersensitive, with a mind worrying about everything and anything. In an empty hand this will not be too bad, but in a full hand the owner's nervous energy will soon become exhausted and ill-health will set in. These people must have adequate rest at all times.

When the Mercury line starts from the head line itself, business acumen will be less instinctive but based more on facts and figures. When the line crosses over the heart line and touches any of the small vertical lines found just slightly to the side of the mount of Mercury, an active interest in the healing arts will be present.

Hand for Business

The modern office equipped with a computer, e-mail facilities, a fax, and a scanner is a second home for these natural salespeople.

GIRDLE OF VENUS AND VIA LASCIVA

The Girdle of Venus is a small semicircular line or series of broken lines running from almost anywhere on the mount of Jupiter through to the mounts of Apollo and/or Mercury above the heart line. The Via Lasciva is a small horizontal or semicircular line that links the base of the mounts of the moon and Venus. Both relate to the degree of sensitivity in the nature of the owner.

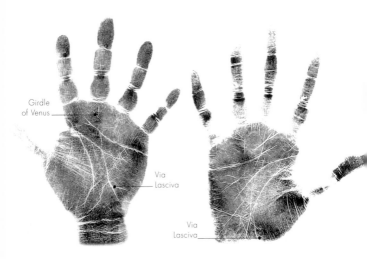

Girdle
of Venus

Via
Lasciva

Via
Lasciva

Both lines in one hand
This print has both a Girdle of Venus and a Via Lasciva. Their combined effect on a character can wreak havoc when the owner lacks or loses personal control and self-discipline.

Via Lasciva
With this line the physical need for stimulation is accentuated and the owner has to find an opportunity for letting off steam from time to time. A straight line could mean an allergy line.

Emotional and physical
The Girdle indicates emotional
sensitivity and the Via Lasciva
shows the amount of physical
sensitivity. They have nothing
to do with each other in a
real sense but they often
seem to work together when
they are both found in the
one hand. Both lines may be
seen together in one hand or
both; in one but not the other;
or they may not be seen at
all, in either hand.

Girdle
of Venus

Via Lasciva

Girdle of Venus and Via Lasciva

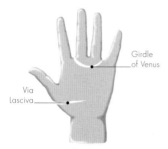

Girdle of Venus

Via Lasciva

Flirtatious

An unbroken Girdle of Venus suggests a flirtatious character.

The Girdle of Venus

This lies along the top of the hand between the first and fourth mounts in one firm or fragmented line, and can be chained or islanded, long or short. It is a measure of the sensitivity in emotional outlook since it is found at the top of the emotional part of the hand.

An unbroken line without interference or faults suggests emotional turmoil and inconsistency in the approach to sex, love, and romance. The overall outlook is usually quite healthy with a good responsive nature but the subject is easily tempted and will be indiscreet, flirtatious, and always ready to tempt fate with an unrealistic relationship.

If on a conic hand, the subjects need stimulation of the senses more than is good for them. On a square hand the owners suffer apprehension when they are challenged, even if they are totally innocent. On a spatulate hand, they are full of nervous excitability, constantly seeking fresh fields to conquer. On the philosophic hand the owners experience a complete loss of control after a project has been concluded. The excitable mixed-hand type cannot stay still for long and will either gossip, gamble, or turn to drink, drugs, or sex when the need arises. The elementary hand rarely has the Girdle, but if it is present, the subject has a foul temper when upset.

If the line is fragmented, emotional intensity is considerably lessened. A short line shows more control but it still represents a very sensitive nature.

The Via Lasciva

This is a small semicircular line that connects the mounts of Venus and Luna. Like the Girdle, it may be fragmented, chained, frayed, or islanded, long or short. In fact, this line varies so much that it may be missed and thought of as a lesser influence marking.

When the line seems to be a simple bridge between these two mounts there is a constant desire for physical stimulation to offset boredom. These people will try anything once in their search to offset this and if they enjoy it, will try it twice. When the line starts from the Venus mount and meanders over to the Luna mount, any physical excesses will be regarded as normal. On a soft square or round hand the owner will take risks to pursue these aims.

Explosive Combination

When these lines are together in the hand expect fireworks. A firm hand lessens the problems while a soft hand adds to them.

THE SUN LINE

The sun or Apollo line is a sister line to the line of fate that can start from almost anywhere but always makes a path toward the base of the third finger. As a rule it usually begins from the head line or between the head and heart lines. It may also start from the heart line or from just above it. It may commence with two short forks and can end the same way, or in the traditionally lucky trident formation.

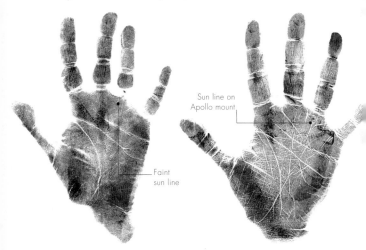

Sun line on
Apollo mount

Faint
sun line

Willing helper

The lightly etched sun line suggests an inwardly happy nature, someone willing to do favors for others provided the owner is initially approached and thanked properly at the end of the exercise.

Practical type

The head and heart lines are aligned in such a way that they reflect a practical and down-to-earth approach to life and all its inherent problems. Little fazes this subject, and the sun line here reflects this attitude.

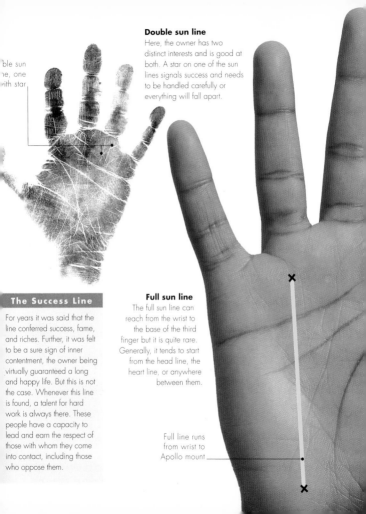

Double sun line
Here, the owner has two distinct interests and is good at both. A star on one of the sun lines signals success and needs to be handled carefully or everything will fall apart.

ble sun
ne, one
vith star

Full sun line
The full sun line can reach from the wrist to the base of the third finger but it is quite rare. Generally, it tends to start from the head line, the heart line, or anywhere between them.

Full line runs from wrist to Apollo mount

The Success Line

For years it was said that the line conferred success, fame, and riches. Further, it was felt to be a sure sign of inner contentment, the owner being virtually guaranteed a long and happy life. But this is not the case. Whenever this line is found, a talent for hard work is always there. These people have a capacity to lead and earn the respect of those with whom they come into contact, including those who oppose them.

The Sun Line

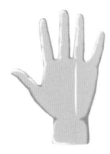

Hard labor
*Those people with a full sun line work
hard to reach their goals in life.*

When the sun line begins at the wrist and goes straight to the mount of Apollo, the subject has to work hard to achieve his or her aims. Any rewards result from the toil itself and are not conferred as a matter of course.

When the sun line begins inside the life line or on the mount of Venus, the family will always be supportive. If the line starts from the life line or just outside it, people with all the necessary influence will always be one step behind the subject.

A line from the mount of Neptune confers counseling talents. Such folk have a gift for dealing with other people, acting as intermediaries, or just listening and allowing others to get things off their chests.

A sun line from the Luna mount allows the subject to enjoy a public career as an entertainer or politician. Both need public approbation and sustained efforts to remain at the top.

A forked start indicates a two-fold edge to the subject's talents and when these people are not in the public eye, a separate interest will be pursued.

When the sun line begins at the head line, extra determination brought about by a strong need to succeed will be evident. In many cases the late starter wins more than those who begin earlier. When the line stops at the head line, it suggests disaster, something from which the subject will never really recover.

When the sun line starts at the heart line, it gives that extra emotional push supporting all the hard work and suggests that all the effort and energy will be a labor of love with little outside help. If the line ends on the heart line, it may involve a fall from grace where everything is lost – possessions, prestige, and the good name and honor of the subject. The cause is often an emotional one.

When the sun line and the fate line merge, all the subject's ambitions should eventually be realized, but only through sheer hard work.

Absent sun line

A hand without a sun line shows an inability to recognize or understand personal limitations. These folk feel that they are immune to any kind of harm and are either unable or unwilling to see that they can fail. Occasionally, there may be a collection of sun lines on a hand showing a multitalented and versatile individual.

Sunny Character

People with a sun line are usually of a cheerful disposition, see pages 178–181.

THE FOUR RINGS

Until very recently only the ring of Solomon, that is, the small circle or line on the mount of the index finger, has been observed by practicing palmists. In the East, this ring has always been thought to confer a sense of duty and obligation with the highest regard for law and order. The other three rings of Saturn, Apollo, and Mercury are rarely seen but if they do appear their contribution to the overall nature must be noted.

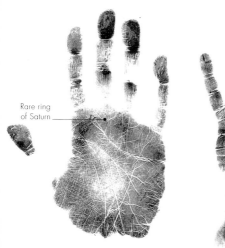

Rare ring of Saturn

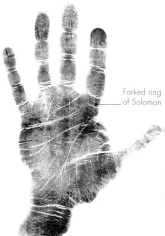

Forked ring of Solomon

Ring of Saturn

This rare ring denies the balance necessary for a well-adjusted character. These subjects consistently fail to achieve their aims, because they cannot seem to get along with anyone at work or play.

Forked Ring of Solomon

When it travels right across the mount in one firm line it indicates an ability to teach. The forked ring on this print shows teaching ability in two separate areas.

Ring of Solomon
The Ring of Solomon crosses the mount of Jupiter, usually from the radial side of the hand to the edge of the skin pattern between the first and second fingers. It does not encircle the base of the index finger as the others do but lies over the mount and more to the top of it.

Ring of Saturn
The ring of Saturn is rare and is usually manifested as a broken line that encircles the base of the middle finger very close to the top of the mount.

Ring of Apollo
The ring of Apollo is a line that travels high on the mount, just below the base of the third finger.

Ring of Mercury
The ring of Mercury encircles the base of the little finger, often in a broken form.

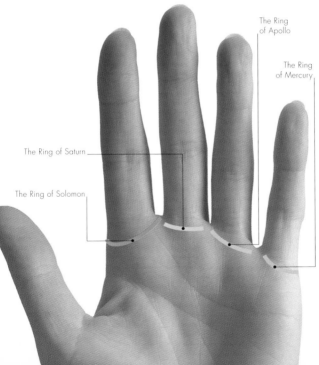

The Ring of Apollo

The Ring of Mercury

The Ring of Saturn

The Ring of Solomon

The Four Rings

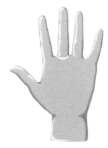

Ring of Saturn
*They are very hard to get to know,
for they do not trust others easily.*

The ring of Solomon

As instructors these folk excel, for they have a way of getting their message over. There is an air of authority that comes with knowledge and causes others to stop and listen. If the line forms a part of a small but clearly defined square on the mount, this teaching ability is emphasized.

A well-formed line indicates social standing, personal prestige with a sense of dignity. Subjects with this mark become magistrates or go into local politics. In due course, they can become the mayor or chair of the local council. Successful legal careers end on the bench as a judge.

There is a deep understanding of people, a natural empathy with others. Successful psychologists often have this line and, if the line of heart starts from it, they make excellent carers.

A fragmented line across the mount indicates a basic, physical approach. The subject has a deeply sensual nature with a strong love of food and drink and enjoys varied indulgences to the full.

The ring of Saturn

This is an extremely rare and basically unfortunate marking. It indicates a lack of spontaneity, difficulty in mixing socially, and it marks the character as something of a lone wolf.

The ring of Apollo

This is another equally unusual mark. When the ring is well made and unbroken, the subject will be known for special creative and artistic talents especially in the entertainment world.

It belongs to those special people who stand head and shoulders above everyone else. However, if they fall, they lose absolutely everything they stood for and will be ostracized by all and sundry. A fragmented or badly made ring of Apollo shows poor taste and equally bad judgment in anything to do with self-presentation.

The ring of Mercury

This is an extremely rare occurrence. Traditionally, it is said to be the mark of a confirmed spinster or bachelor. There is no inclination to marry or live with a partner of the opposite sex. This is not a sign of homosexuality – they simply cannot get along with each other.

In the hands of businesspeople, it confers commercial acumen and a drive to achieve power and wealth, often at the expense of others.

Shady Dealings

A fragmented Mercury ring shows an inclination to get involved in questionable dealings, especially concerning money.

LOVE, TRAVEL, AND FRUSTRATION

Love and marriage will be shown by the lines on the outer percussion side of the hand, above the end of the heart line just below the Mercury finger. The size of the hand and Luna mount is an indicator of those with the travel bug, especially if there is a horizontal line across from the outer edge of the hand. Small horizontal lines on the lower phalanges of the fingers are a sign of irritability and frustration.

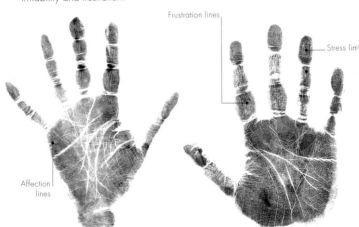

Frustration lines

Stress line

Affection lines

Affection lines

Horizontal lines from the Mercury mount were used to record marriage, and the vertical lines rising up from them children. Horizontal lines are now treated as serious love affairs or romances that have left their mark and vertical lines refer to close mutual friends involved in making it all work.

Stress, strain, and frustration

Serious but temporary strain and low physical reserves are shown when the top phalanges of all the fingers show horizontal "white lines" across them. They often appear at the end of a trying day or after long periods of concentration. Vertical lines on the lower phalanges indicate frustration.

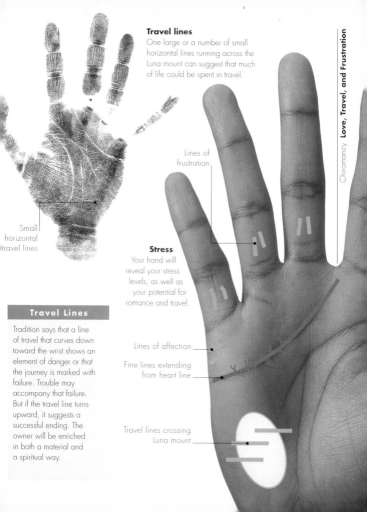

Travel lines
One large or a number of small horizontal lines running across the Luna mount can suggest that much of life could be spent in travel.

Lines of frustration

Stress
Your hand will reveal your stress levels, as well as your potential for romance and travel.

Small horizontal travel lines

Lines of affection

Fine lines extending from heart line

Travel lines crossing Luna mount

Travel Lines

Tradition says that a line of travel that curves down toward the wrist shows an element of danger or that the journey is marked with failure. Trouble may accompany that failure. But if the travel line turns upward, it suggests a successful ending. The owner will be enriched in both a material and a spiritual way.

Recognizng Attachment, Travel, and Frustration Lines

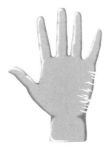

Travel bug
Horizontal lines from the outer edge indicate restlessness or a desire to travel.

Attachment lines

The darker these lines, the stronger the basis of such a liaison. The first small bar from the outer edge just above the heart line may only reach a half inch (one centimeter) long before it merges with it. This records the owner's first love, often the most memorable affair, regarded with much fondness.

A line from the Luna mount that joins with the fate line indicates a new partnership of equal strength, not always marriage, but a warm and human friendship, someone who can always be relied on through thick and thin.

Travel lines

The wider and bigger the hand, the less routine attracts, and as a rule there will be a large mount of Luna to support this. When it is large, firm, and quite prominent, it indicates people who have a need to keep on the move. The owners are restive and need to travel even if only locally. They live life on the run.

A bold, clearly etched horizontal line from the outer edge of the hand is an indication of travel, often overseas and with a chance of living there for a while. If the line is faint or has other minor lines with it, the subject will travel extensively overseas. Smaller, short lines can mean travel, but shorter journeys, such as those of a courier.

If a travel line cuts through the life line, an element of danger associated with water is suggested. However,

when this interpretation was first
introduced, travel overseas could only
have been by ship, because airplanes
had not been invented at that time.
Today, I would include danger by
both sea and air.

Lines of irritation
and frustration

When they appear on all the fingers the
owner cannot cope with stress at all. If
vertical lines are also seen running up
the length of the fingers, stress of a
substantial order will affect the subject.
If the basal phalanges look fluffed or
podgy, the issue will be aggravated, in
which case check the head line. If it has
a fluffy appearance, mental stress will
also be involved.

White Flecking

White flecking of the nails is another symptom
of strain, perhaps more nervous in origin. If the
flecking fades away, the tensions will ease
and, with it, any irritability.

FAMILY, LOYALTY, AND RASCETTES

The family ring links the second and third phalange of the thumb and is the only "ring" without the cutting-off effect. It is nearly always poorly formed, fragmented, or chained in its appearance. The loyalty line may be either one small line or a series of lines that cross the upper part of the mount of Venus or the old mount of Mars positive. The rascettes, or bracelets, run across the inside of the wrist just below the palm. Usually there are one, two, or three present but there can be more.

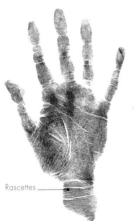

Rascettes

Family ring

Rascettes
The bracelets or rascettes are often ignored by student and professional alike. Travel lines that reach down into the top ring have long been considered traditionally to mark eventful journeys for good or ill.

The family ring
The family ring shows solidarity with the family if reasonably well formed. Often, it is a chained affair that suggests certain interfamily relationships blow hot and cold. A fairly common sign found in many hands.

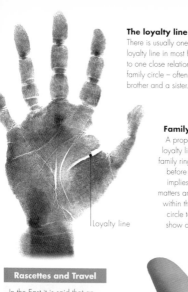

The loyalty line

There is usually one strongly etched loyalty line in most hands referring to one close relationship within the family circle – often between a brother and a sister.

Loyalty line

Family matters

A properly formed loyalty line from the family ring that stops before the life line implies that family matters are kept well within the domestic circle to present a show of solidarity.

In the East it is said that an influence line originating from one of the rascettes to the Luna mount shows a love of travel and more than one line is a sure sign that travel attracts, but one of the lines must start from the lowest bracelet. A square touching on one of the influence lines is a sign of protection for as long as the journey takes. An island suggests trouble. A star at the end of any of the lines presages a successful finale to a journey.

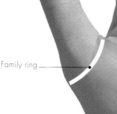

Loyalty line

Family ring

The rascettes or bracelets

The Family Ring, Loyalty Line, and the Rascettes

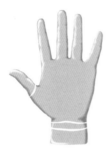

Close relations
Longevity and family ties are revealed by the rascettes and the family ring.

The family ring

In some hands the family ring has a very deep, emphatic look to it; in others it looks almost indecipherable. Close family ties are shown by a well-marked line, while little love is lost for close family if it is virtually nonexistent.

If the ring is well marked at the top inner side of the thumb but seems weaker at the bottom, it suggests all was well in the early years, but that now this all has gone by the board.

The loyalty line

These may originate from the family ring and reach the life line, which shows a very strong sense of loyalty to or a need for one of the family. It can be either of the parents, a brother, or a sister.

If the line begins at the family ring this closeness will be emphasized. If there is more than one line and they all start from the family ring, few people will penetrate the inner domestic circle. The family's good name will be zealously guarded at all times. If all the lines remain inside the life line, all problems will stay within the family to be solved by them.

The rascettes

Traditionally, they are linked with longevity by Eastern palm reading but in the West there is little evidence to support this. However, a few nonagenarians have had three or four well-marked bracelets and, in a small number of cases, the life line ended only after it had passed through the top one.

When in a woman's hand the first rascette arches into the base of the hand, it suggests difficulties with the urinogenital system and is associated with bladder or menstrual problems. It makes sense to have a look at the hands of young girls, for if this occurs and is seen early enough it might save some adolescent difficulties. If the next bracelet also rises, these problems will be aggravated.

This arching of the bracelet can sometimes be seen in the hand of a man and suggests prostate or similar problems. Traditionally, it was always thought the bracelets were associated with travel or a desire to do so. Good, well-formed bracelets that cross the wrist without interference suggest the owner does not suffer from travel sickness.

Wealth and Success

In the Eastern palm reading tradition, four or more rascettes promised wealth and success together with a long and happy life.

THE LINE OF INTUITION
People with a natural prescience, the ability to be guided by an inner sixth sense, usually have a pronounced mount of Neptune. As a rule, this gift manifests itself by the owner just "knowing" something is about to happen or about an event that has occurred miles away. For a more practical approach to this kind of second sight, "awareness," or plain old-fashioned instinct, look for the line of intuition.

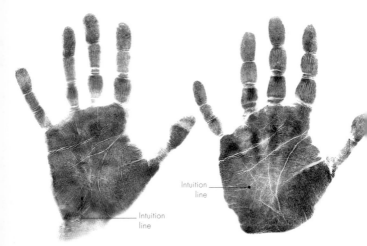

Intuition line

Intuition line

Low-set line
This quite low-set intuition line suggests the owner puts his or her natural prescience to a practical use and may be able to see the answer to a question before the other party has finished detailing it.

Perceptive
The owner of this active hand makes good use of his or her intuition line by seemingly always "knowing" the right thing to do or say at just the right time.

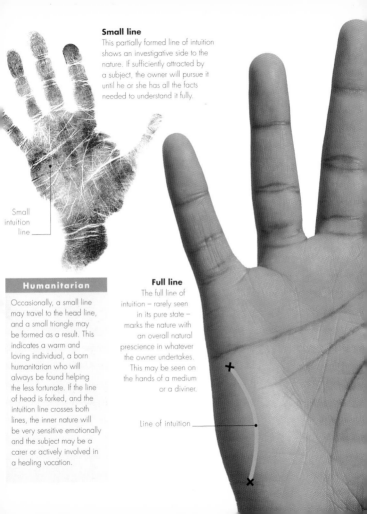

Small line
This partially formed line of intuition shows an investigative side to the nature. If sufficiently attracted by a subject, the owner will pursue it until he or she has all the facts needed to understand it fully.

Small intuition line

Humanitarian

Occasionally, a small line may travel to the head line, and a small triangle may be formed as a result. This indicates a warm and loving individual, a born humanitarian who will always be found helping the less fortunate. If the line of head is forked, and the intuition line crosses both lines, the inner nature will be very sensitive emotionally and the subject may be a carer or actively involved in a healing vocation.

Full line
The full line of intuition – rarely seen in its pure state – marks the nature with an overall natural prescience in whatever the owner undertakes. This may be seen on the hands of a medium or a diviner.

Line of intuition

The Line of Intuition

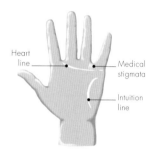

Healing power
An intuition line with the medical stigmata shows a talent for healing.

The line of intuition is a small, often badly fragmented line that can start from anywhere on the Luna mount near the edge of the hand and rise upward. It gently curves deeper into the mount of the moon and ends almost anywhere on the mount of Mercury.

It is rare to see it as a continuous line, for it can look like a collection of small influence lines, or appear chained or islanded throughout. When it does form one continuous line, it shows an innate love of investigative or research work, someone who has the patience to sift endlessly through piles of information and reach satisfactory conclusions. People like this have usually had a good education, which is reflected in the way they express themselves.

They "absorb" rather than learn in conventional ways, and have a fluency of thought, of knowing things without being aware of it. Because of this these people eventually find occult studies are for them and this helps to develop their gifts even more.

With suitable training they can become astrologers, palmists, Tarot readers, or whatever. Mediums often have some semblance of this mark in their left hands, showing the gift is inherited and the predictive arts come naturally, and if the line makes a triangle with the fate line and the head line, it is said to be the traditional sign of a seer. Hypnotism is also another suitable field of endeavor for their talents.

The more faults on the line, the weaker the owner's talent. An occasional flash of brilliance, nothing more. Generally, when the whole line or a good part of it is present, the owners have a gift for coaxing animals to obey their commands.

When the line is on both hands, the subject tends to gravitate toward occult matters and often makes a good medium, with proper training of course. If the medical stigmata are also present, the power of healing is a possibility, aided with a strongly intuitive insight. With a creative curve and a sloping head line, he or she may even be a psychic artist.

The Medical Stigmata

The medical stigmata are a small series of four or five short vertical lines slightly to the inner side of the mount of Mercury, just above the heart line. They indicate an interest in medical matters, fringe medicine, and anything to do with healing.

In addition, there may be some evidence of mild hypochondria sometimes connected with stress and strain. The subject keeps to a preset daily routine and will not vary it one iota. Diet and health may also be involved.

Sometimes these lines may reflect dental problems, especially if very deeply etched and very close together.

PRACTICAL
PALM READING

All the basic principles for reading hands have now been set out. You are now ready to put what you have learned into practice. You have all you need to start to practice and you must keep at it all the time, for this study relies on continual practical expertise. ⮕ Don't be afraid of making a mistake – we all do it, no matter what we do for a living, so why should you worry? Try not to seize on one special mark and concentrate on the gifts it may confer. There may be other marks present in the hand, not previously noticed, that do not tie in with what you say. ⮕ People are almost always willing to let you look at their hands, because this is a fascinating study and, what is more, it is always about their favorite subject – themselves.

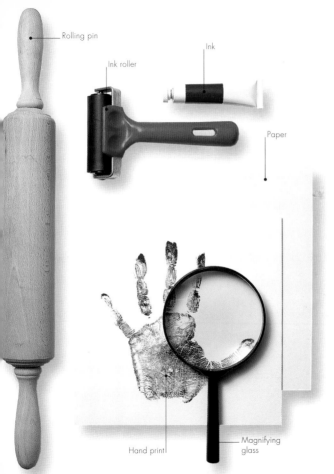

Rolling pin

Ink roller

Ink

Paper

Hand print

Magnifying glass

Before You Start

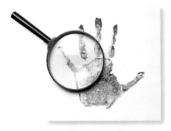

Close inspection
A powerful magnifying glass is essential for scrutinizing lines in detail.

In the East, many palmists follow a set ritual prior to reading hands. Often, the client is expected to attend at dawn, for many believe a palmist's gifts are then at their highest. The mind is not cluttered with matters that have occurred earlier and is free to concentrate.

Very few of these masters use a magnifying glass but they insist that the hands must first be washed, patted dry, scented, then placed on a cushion ready for the reading. Both hands are read and, because of their knowledge, these palmists also use a form of astrology for dating events from the past and in the future. Few Western palmists have this type of training and many frown on using other disciplines like this.

In the West, hand reading does not involve astrology. There is no need to supply a birth date or give your name. When the reading is to be taken from hand prints, all a good palmist needs is the sex and age of the client. If you supply other data the palmist may then be able to consult astrology and/or numerology books, which is an unfair advantage and not real hand reading.

The time of the reading is irrelevant. Make sure that you seat the subject in a comfortable chair and have both hands placed underneath a bright light. You really must have a set of good, clear hand prints by you at all times, and in special cases take fresh prints prior to each session.

You will need a powerful magnifying glass, a small ruler, a pen or pencil, and a pair of compasses. Some people like to have tape recordings made of the interview, so a reliable recorder should be available.

Keeping records

Many people consult on a regular basis
so it is wise to take proper notes every
time. A short reading is often only
concerned with a current problem for
which the client may have specifically
wanted advice. A full reading, with all
the trimmings and an eventual written
(typed) report, could easily take several
sessions – the tape recorder then
becomes necessary, so remember to
maintain your records religiously.

Keeping a good record system
is necessary because over a period
of time any changes in the hands,
however small, will soon become
apparent. A box file holding cards 3 x
5 inches (7.5 x 12.5cm) is ideal for
this exercise. One should note these
changes and any other features of
analysis that may be special to that
particular client.

Making Hand Prints

For additional information on making and
reading palm prints, see pages 46–49.

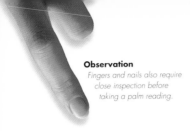

Observation
*Fingers and nails also require
close inspection before
taking a palm reading.*

HAND EXERCISES
We will assume you have obtained all the equipment that has been recommended and your client has entered the room. You will need to ascertain a few important details before you examine the hands. It is always important to make pre-interview notes, so that you may clear up a problem that may have arisen before you start or, during analysis, to help clarify other matters.

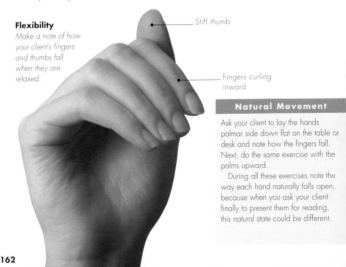

Flexibility
*Make a note of how
your client's fingers
and thumbs fall
when they are
relaxed.*

Stiff thumb

Fingers curling
inward

Natural Movement

Ask your client to lay the hands palmar side down flat on the table or desk and note how the fingers fall. Next, do the same exercise with the palms upward.

During all these exercises note the way each hand naturally falls open, because when you ask your client finally to present them for reading, this natural state could be different.

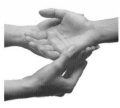

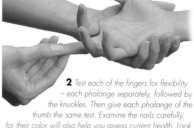

1 You must now physically feel the hands to see if they are hard or soft to the touch. Hard hands imply energy and activity, soft hands do not. Check all the mounts to see if they feel fleshy or bony, thick or thin. Test the mouse mount at the back of a hand because it is important you are aware of the current state of health of the client.

2 Test each of the fingers for flexibility – each phalange separately, followed by the knuckles. Then give each phalange of the thumb the same test. Examine the nails carefully, for their color will also help you assess current health. Look at the fingertips to see if there are any white lines suggesting stress and strain. Note how the hands feel – how warm, hot, or cold, and dry or moist they are, considering the temperature and how long they have been in the room.

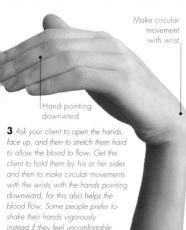

Make circular movement with wrist

Hand pointing downward

3 Ask your client to open the hands, face up, and then to stretch them hard to allow the blood to flow. Get the client to hold them by his or her sides and then to make circular movements with the wrists with the hands pointing downward, for this also helps the blood flow. Some people prefer to shake their hands vigorously instead if they feel uncomfortable with circular movement.

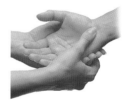

4 Hold one hand at the wrist, with the palmar side toward you, and squeeze it hard for a few seconds and then do the same with the other hand afterward. This exercise makes the lines of the hand seem a little more prominent for a short while and gives you an opportunity to assess them, albeit briefly.

Hand Analysis

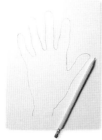

Outline
*Draw an outline of the hand to help
you assess size and shape.*

Y ou will have already gained
quite a lot of knowledge about
the type of hands that you are
about to analyze by the time the client
settles down in front of you and opens
the hands for your first appraisal.

You will have tested the hands for
flexibility, noted the current state of
health, and assessed their size (in
relation to build), as well as noticed
if the client is left- or right-handed.

By noting the way in which the
hands and fingers fall open you will
have discovered certain personality

traits: whether the client is tight-fisted
or open-hearted, naturally open and
friendly or worried and suspicious.

The size of the hands will tell you
how to relay your findings and how
to talk to the person: in great detail for
those with large hands or when the
fingers are longer than the palm; for the
small-handed, with fingers shorter than
the palm, you may gloss over details
and give the wider picture.

Dialogue

The first thing to do is to assess the
type of hand and note if it is basically
square or round. There may be an
extension to the basic shape and you
must hone your assessment accordingly.

Once you are satisfied you have
described the qualities of the hand you
must not be afraid to ask questions in
order to clarify details. Invite the client
to ask questions; establish a dialogue
as early as you can in any interview.

While you have been talking you will
have noticed the lines and, at the very
least, decided if the client has a full,

empty, or average hand. Plenty of lines criss-crossing all over the palm warn you to moderate what you say, because the client's imagination will be working overtime during the session.

The empty hand is not that easy either and may produce monosyllabic responses that are hard to interpret. The average hand is helpful until you touch on a sensitive matter, then the client will go quiet. In due course, experience will teach you this and you will be able to help the client more easily.

The last, but by no means least, step is to examine the finger and palm prints for the part they play in the personality before you. Every time you read a pair of hands you gain experience, feel more confident, and more able to help those who have come to consult you.

Be Patient and Listen

While you will want to demonstrate your new powers, you must always be prepared to be patient. Always find out what your subjects want to say as much as listening to what they actually do say. You will learn a lot about people, and yourself as well.

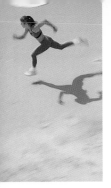

Leaps and bounds
Palms that are firm to the touch are signs of a strong constitution.

HEALTH AND THE HANDS

Test the hand physically for firmness and resilience, especially in the center of the palm. When the center of the palm feels firm, the current health is good, but if it feels soft in the right hand and firm in the left, what ill-health may be troubling the owner will be short-lived. If the life line swings out into the palm, most illness is easily thrown off and the constitution is strong.

The mouse
Get the subject to make a fist so you can check the small mount at the back of the hand and the thumb – the mouse.

A firm mouse shows good health

Extroversion/Introversion

Extrovert people, the hale and hearty types, and introverted folk, the withdrawn and quiet sort, are assessed from the amount of space between the lines of heart and head, the "Great Quadrangle."

When the gap is wide the owner is much more physically active, outgoing, and level-headed. The wider this space the more this is so. When the gap is narrow, the nature is much less outgoing, someone who lets the world pass by.

When these two types suffer temporary spells of poor health, the extrovert types will be edgy, irritable, and show their anger physically, while the introverted look worse than they actually are and may even enjoy not being well in order to elicit some sympathy.

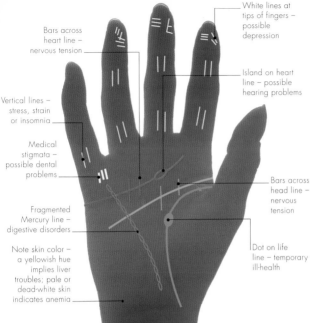

White lines at tips of fingers – possible depression

Bars across heart line – nervous tension

Island on heart line – possible hearing problems

Vertical lines – stress, strain or insomnia

Medical stigmata – possible dental problems

Bars across head line – nervous tension

Fragmented Mercury line – digestive disorders

Dot on life line – temporary ill-health

Note skin color – a yellowish hue implies liver troubles; pale or dead-white skin indicates anemia

Special Marks and Your Health

An island on the life line indicates poor health. On the heart line it shows hearing problems or heart trouble.

The need for an operation may be shown by a small triangle, cross, or a square on the life line about

two-thirds of the way down. It does not mean the subject will have to have one, only that it may become necessary.

Chaining on the heart line indicates vascular disorders, on the life line – a poor constitution.

General Health and Vitality

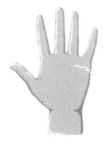

Worrier
A fine tracery of fragmented lines is a sign of hypersensitivity.

If the mount of Venus is soft to the touch and the line of life seems to hug around the base as if restricting its development, the owner does not have very good recovery powers. A soft hand shows indolence and a lazy streak, so a chance to take time off work, even for the common cold, will be seized with both hands, so to speak.

Between the middle of the base of the third and fourth fingers just above the heart line, three or four small vertical lines show possible dental problems. They do not cause trouble when they occur, but simply show a predisposition.

Stress and strain

When the two bottom phalanges of all the fingers have vertical lines on them the subject may have trouble sleeping at night. If there is a full hand, it shows that the owner has trouble switching off. The vertical lines often appear on those who work shift patterns.

The possible causes for depression may be located at a number of places in the palm. The full hand is often one sign, because the mind is never still and the imagination runs wild at the slightest excuse. White lines at the tips of the fingers are also a sign. Vertical lines may reflect a temporary period of hormonal imbalance, while horizontal ones are the result of burning the candle at both ends – the owner has tapped into the nervous energy reserves far more than is good for that person.

Digestive system

Digestive disorders are shown when the Mercury line is present but in a fragmented, chained, or islanded formation. Small influence lines that

rise up from the middle of the zone
of Mars toward the base of the third
finger indicate internal problems
connected with the digestive system.

A very soft-to-the-touch base phalange
of the index finger shows that the owner
must be careful with what he or she eats
and if the allergy line is seen at the base
of the palm this will be emphasized.

Hearing problems

Hearing difficulties are illustrated by a
distinct island in the heart line below the
middle finger. To see how bad this is or
may become, check the flexibility of the
tip of the little finger. A stiff tip suggests
a check-up is advisable, while a flexible
tip shows a temporary matter, but it is
still worth having hearing checked.

A Word of Caution

Unless you have medical training you must not
make statements as though you have. Untold
damage can be caused by a wrong word at
such times. If you think there are problems,
you should quietly and tactfully advise your
client to see a doctor or have a checkup.

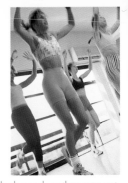

Health conscious
The condition of the nails can tell you a great deal about a person's state of health and the lifestyle they lead.

NAILS AND HEALTH

Whether we are trained observers or not, very often the first thing we notice with most hands is the state of their nails. They may be well kept or look good, or they may not. Women's nails, and even some men's, may have nail polish, which is unhelpful in assessing the current state of health. An analysis of the nails can show mineral deficiency, nervous tension and strain, and vascular problems.

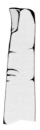

Dished nails
Dished (concave) nails usually imply a glandular problem, probably through poor blood supply or nutritional deficiency.

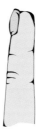

Bulbous nail
The bulbous, curved nail is known as the Hippocratic nail, and is a clear symptom of chest or respiratory problems such as those caused by heavy smoking.

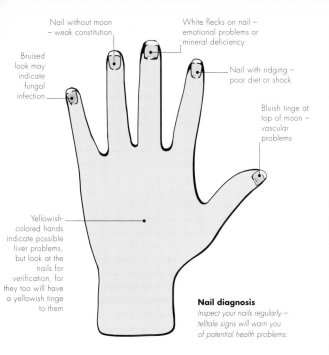

Nail without moon
– weak constitution

White flecks on nail –
emotional problems or
mineral deficiency

Bruised
look may
indicate
fungal
infection

Nail with ridging –
poor diet or shock

Bluish tinge at
top of moon –
vascular
problems

Yellowish-colored hands
indicate possible
liver problems,
but look at the
nails for
verification, for
they too will have
a yellowish tinge
to them

Nail diagnosis
*Inspect your nails regularly –
telltale signs will warn you
of potential health problems.*

Nail Shapes and Health

A shell-shaped
nail shows generally
poor health and
hypersensitivity.

A talon-shaped
nail indicates
a nutritionally
poor diet.

Those with large
square nails have a
predisposition to
suppress problems.

Analysis of the Nails

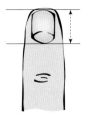

Nail growth
It takes around six months for a nail to grow from root to tip, so any marks on the nail can be dated easily.

The nail is made up from a hard protein called keratin and takes about six months to grow out from the root in a continuous growth process, and any marks that appear on the nail, such as white flecks, bars, or other damage, can thus be dated easily. However, this does not refer to the horizontal or vertical ridging that suddenly appears because of certain illnesses such as stress or strain. When this happens it indicates weakness involving glandular, organic, or endocrine imbalance. As a rule this makes the subject tired and irritable.

When white specks are found on bitten nails it suggests that some emotional trouble or a psychological problem is worrying the individual and consequently affecting his or her health. With horizontal and longitudinal ridging the cause may be a recent accident, emotional shock, or simply a poor diet. Each nail should display a well-formed, clear moon at the base, but where none are seen a temporary problem affecting the constitution is indicated.

Nail shapes

The short nail always shows a worrying nature; the larger square one, people who are inclined to bottle things up and exert too much emotional control.

People with narrow nails are rather delicate and tire easily. A slight bluish color at the top of the moon suggests a vascular problem.

Shell-shaped nails always refer to a state of rundown health that often sets in after a shock to the system, while the talon type suggests poor attention to diet, which will result in health problems.

Those with filbert (hazelnut-shaped) nails live on their nervous energy reserves far more than is good for them.

Dished or concave nails show that the owner is suffering glandular problems possibly through poor blood flow or eating all the wrong things at the wrong time. They are often dull and listless people. The bulbous nail – the Hippocratic nail – is a sure sign of respiratory problems, probably caused through heavy smoking.

Any predisposition to catching sore throats, colds, or serious respiratory ailments will be indicated by a bulbous nail on the first finger, which can show the early stages. If the other nails start to take on a similar shape or the head line begins in a chained or islanded fashion, the troubles will be aggravated.

Small or Large Nails?

People who have large nails tend to lead a more peaceful, balanced, and expansive life. Those folk with small nails have critical nature and, perhaps, a slightly more restricted approach to life.

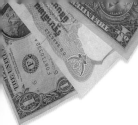

In the money
Signs of material wealth can be detected in the hands – you may even strike lucky and win the lottery.

WEALTH

There are two types of wealth: inner personal happiness and financial. When you meet someone, especially for the first time, you tend to assess them by their actions, and a quick look at their hands will help you confirm this assessment. The wider the fingers spread and the hand opens, the more open and friendly the nature especially if there is a Sun line in the hand.

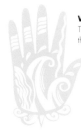

Water hand
These folk flourish where they are able to exercise their creative powers fully in the entertainment or beauty industries.

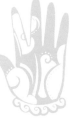

Air hand
Air hands enjoy money and possessions but they do like to work for them so they may boast that they did it their way.

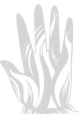

Fire hand
The Fire hand enjoys and luxuriates in material wealth. These people must have the best if they are to have anything at all.

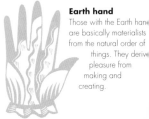

Earth hand
Those with the Earth hand are basically materialists from the natural order of things. They derive pleasure from making and creating.

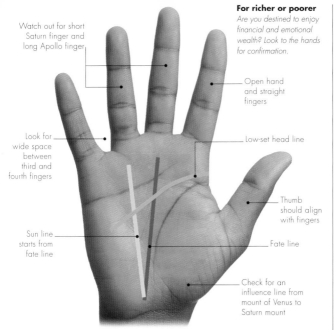

Watch out for short Saturn finger and long Apollo finger

For richer or poorer

Are you destined to enjoy financial and emotional wealth? Look to the hands for confirmation.

Open hand and straight fingers

Look for wide space between third and fourth fingers

Low-set head line

Thumb should align with fingers

Sun line starts from fate line

Fate line

Check for an influence line from mount of Venus to Saturn mount

Special Marks and Your Wealth

A trident at the end of the fate line has always been recognized as the sign of material success but we are beginning to wander into the realms of old-fashioned fortunetelling.

A sun line, once known as the fortune line, that starts from the fate line is always helpful especially when it ends with a star. A star at the end of the old-style

marriage lines on the Mercury mount just above the heart line has always been interpreted as meaning a "good" marriage, implying status and material success.

Wealth

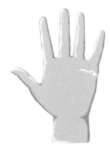

Alignment
When a person holds out the hand, note the angle of the thumb in relation to the fingers.

An "open" hand almost always represents an open personality, the person who enjoys meeting and being with others. These people shine in company and will make sure that everyone enjoys themselves, helping a party go with a swing. They make good, reliable friends.

Their hands are nearly always held open; the fingers are straight, not curled inward like a claw, as if covering the palm from general view. The thumb will almost always align with the fingers in these cases.

When people show you their hands they tend to hold them palms upward, in which case note the thumb. It will look like another finger and in line with them, or it will be at angle as if it opposes them. When it lines up along with the fingers so you can see all of the inner part quite clearly, your subject has little to hide and is the life and soul of any social gathering.

If there is a wide space between the third and fourth fingers, they will be open and free with their affections and can be generous if the mood takes them.

Wealth signs

There is no straightforward sign, mark, or line that indicates monetary wealth. But there are a number of features that indicate the possibility of acquiring wealth. However, an influence line that runs from the mount of Venus to the Saturn mount suggests inheritance coming from within the family circle.

The trident, a very rare sign in Western palm reading, always presages material wealth especially when on the mounts of Jupiter or Mercury. On the first mount it shows that ambitions will be realized; if we want money and position and are prepared to work for them, they will come. When on the fourth, finer mount, it shows that good commercial sense will realize just rewards in much the same way.

A kind, generous, and understanding nature is always indicated by a low-set line of heart. The lower the line lies in the palm, the warmer that nature. This is a sure-fire indication of an innate understanding of the problems of others. They have a good sense of values and will share good fortune quite readily.

Gambling

When the head line curls up toward the Mercury mount it shows ruthless pursuit of material success. A rare sign, it has been seen in the hands of self-made millionaires. Tradition suggests a cross on the mount of Jupiter shows unearned money will come your way. Always look at the middle finger of any intended partner. A Saturn finger shorter than the first and third fingers shows a gambling nature but, be warned, such folk are not reliable, except if or when they win.

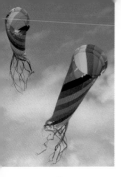

Harmony

A happy and harmonious working or loving relationship with another person may depend on the compatibility of your hands.

HAPPINESS

As far as palm reading is concerned precious little has been discussed with regard to inner, personal happiness. However, there are several indicators to look out for on the hand. Certain hand types are more compatible than others, so note these guidelines to ensure that you get the most from your relationships.

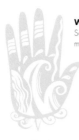

Water hand

Somewhat sensitive to all manner of atmospheres, these people flourish best where they are able to express their creative powers to the full.

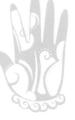

Air hand

The Air hand types are likely to get a lot of pleasure from exercising their brains with puzzles that really challenge them.

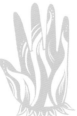

Fire hand

People with Fire hands like to be kept busy and derive their satisfaction from starting, pursuing, and completing a project under their own steam.

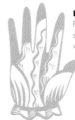

Earth hand

People with the Earth shape prefer to create with their hands and obtain great inner satisfaction from the end result.

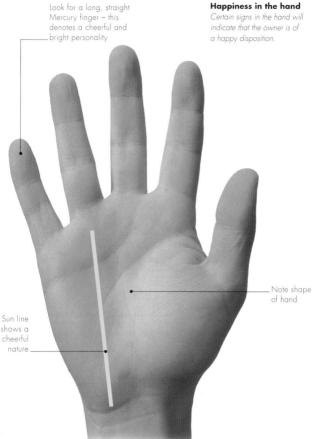

Look for a long, straight Mercury finger – this denotes a cheerful and bright personality

Happiness in the hand
Certain signs in the hand will indicate that the owner is of a happy disposition.

Note shape of hand

Sun line shows a cheerful nature

Happiness

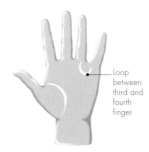

Loop between third and fourth finger

Loop of humor

A loop between the third and fourth fingers indicates happiness.

When the Mercury finger is long and straight, at least up to the first phalangeal joint of the index finger, the owners will always demonstrate their inner happiness and sense of humor in the way they go about their daily lives.

These people have magnetic personalities and light up the room when they enter. With a soft palm they will probably be gigglers to go with their infectious character, people who appreciate the good life and the odd funny story.

Between the third and fourth fingers a little loop is sometimes seen in the skin pattern and is a very good sign of a happy inner nature. If it inclines toward the Apollo mount, an innate sense of the ridiculous and fun is evident.

Compatibility

Different hand types can mix and get on very well with other people with whom they must work or socialize, almost as well as they get along with the same kind of personality. For example, two square-handed people can get along well together because they have the same goals, but they may well bog each other down with the rules.

A square and a conic hand working together will find their strengths in allowing the other to bring his or her respective talents to the table – one is a realist, the other creative. A square and a spatulate hand find equal motivation since they both like to get things done.

The square hand with the philosophic may not be adventurous, but they can and do achieve. Two conic hands will either have a good rapport or they will be touchy and moody and nothing will get done. A conic hand tries to work with a philosophic type, but this is a meeting of the rational and irrational and, while opposites attract... .

Conic and spatulate hands produce a high-powered problem-solving duo but impatience may cause them not to keep their promises. And when two philosophic-handed people work together they create excellent results but are just never satisfied with anything. Philosophic and spatulate hands live and work on a tightrope, and fireworks are always likely.

Two spatulates will probably work until they exhaust each other, for they will both do anything to win the point, but they will be happy while together.

The Sun Line

The sun line is always a sure sign of a bright inner nature with a pleasant overall disposition. Owners lead and inspire through sheer industry. However, like everyone else, they have their off moments as well.

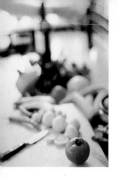

CASE STUDY: THE COOK

Cooking is an art form; one must have an instinctive flair for it. It involves hard work physically, a knowledge of what to buy and when, and a good knowledge of dietary requirements. Presentation also comes into play here; it is one thing to prepare, but quite another to serve it all up.

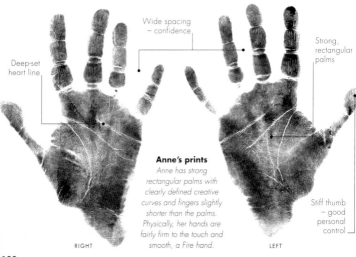

Wide spacing – confidence

Deep-set heart line

Strong, rectangular palms

Anne's prints
Anne has strong rectangular palms with clearly defined creative curves and fingers slightly shorter than the palms. Physically, her hands are fairly firm to the touch and smooth, a Fire hand.

Stiff thumb – good personal control

RIGHT   LEFT

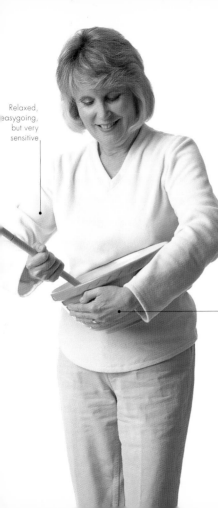

Relaxed, easygoing, but very sensitive

Fire hand

Anne has a Fire hand, which suggests a happy-go-lucky, active type full of ideas and not afraid to put them into practice. She may not always see the point of an argument, is a little less perceptive than most at times, and can be vague occasionally, but she generally comes down to earth just at the right time – typical of a Fire hand. But, perhaps it is because of her thumbs, which are a trifle stiff and unyielding, suggesting good personal control.

Puts good ideas into practice

Anne the Cook

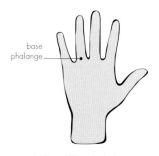

base phalange

Enlarged basal phalanges
Anne's enlarged basal phalanges indicate her talent for cooking.

In both of Anne's hands the head and life lines start apart from each other with a only a few influence marks to link them and this helps boost her personal confidence. She will take a chance and instinctively knows just how far she can go or let others go. The wide spacing between her fingers shows a love of independence but her quite deeply set heart line says otherwise; she is emotionally dependent, so occasionally there is a clash of needs and wants.

Each finger has enlarged base phalanges, especially the indexes, and this is always a sign of someone who not only knows good food but also how to use it to maximum effect. It also means proficiency in food preparation skills from the early years.

Creative and sensitive

In her right hand there is a slightly bowed head line, once again showing an interest in the creative arts rather than the sciences, the best way in which to express herself. She enjoys being with people, and makes her other talents – the arts of sewing and making clothes and floristry – look so simple. The line of head in the left hand suggests a more practical approach.

Her life line in the right hand sweeps out into the palm while the line in her left hand is a little tighter. In her earlier years she had to be careful in her self-expression and natural enthusiasm for life. However, as she has grown and matured she has gradually released those tensions.

She is far more easygoing now but still very sensitive. There is a stronger Girdle of Venus in the right hand than in the left. She will only go so far before she quietens down and changes and, although those close to her may not notice, others might.

The middle and third fingers incline toward each other in both hands. She is quite careful about her immediate concerns and needs constant reassurance that she is secure and has little to worry about.

Although she has a quite firm fate line in her left hand, in her right hand it is almost nonexistent. Whatever hopes she may have had in early years have all but faded. However, both hands show the loop of serious intent, in the skin pattern between the middle and third fingers, which means that she still holds on to some of her ambitions.

Other Case Studies

For other case studies, see also Phil on pages 186–189 and Alec on pages 206–209.

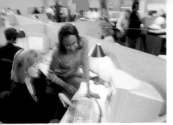

Computer skills

Phil is able to assess how data for a project should be input into a computer to generate results, and then how to present them to those who need to know.

CASE STUDY: THE ACCOUNTANT

Phil's work involves different analysis and audit procedures. He has to be continually aware of and advise on organization and method. He has to keep up to date on taxation and interpret and verify precisely what is needed both by the government and by his company. He also has to set up and maintain financial records of everything that goes on within that company and be aware of market trends in case he is asked to cost potential business ventures.

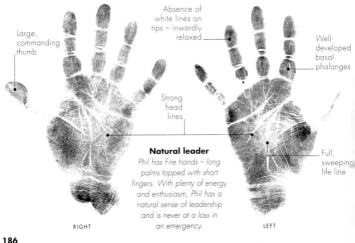

Large, commanding thumb

Absence of white lines on tips – inwardly relaxed

Well-developed basal phalanges

Strong head lines

Natural leader

Phil has Fire hands – long palms topped with short fingers. With plenty of energy and enthusiasm, Phil has a natural sense of leadership and is never at a loss in an emergency.

Full, sweeping life line

RIGHT

LEFT

Requirements of the job

The basic requirements here are for a first-class education, perception, intelligence, and perseverance. He needs to have clear self-expression and give plenty of attention to detail. He must grasp facts quickly and work well with people from all walks of life.

With the advent of the personal computer he has had to learn about them as well. Fortunately, he developed a flair for systems analysis work.

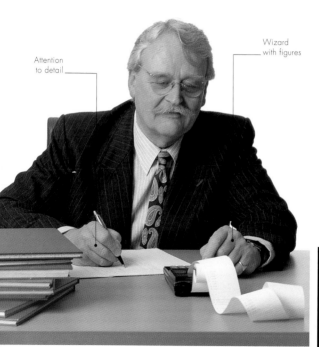

Wizard with figures

Attention to detail

Phil the Accountant

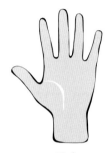

Tireless
Phil's full sweeping life lines show a capacity for sustained hard work.

The first thing one might notice in Phil's palm is the strength of both head lines. When he has to he will blot out all unnecessary matters to concentrate on the problems of the moment. At such times he may appear ruthless but the job has to come first.

He puts his company requirements first and foremost every time. He has large commanding thumbs; you must not argue with Phil unless you have all the right facts, otherwise he will clearly explain a need for accuracy and attention to detail in very succinct terms.

Independent and hard working

Phil has a full sweeping line of life on both hands, which indicates the capacity to work flat out for long stretches at a time. His large palms are firm to the touch with all the mounts in the right proportion.

There is a slight need for Phil to operate independently, which is shown by the little finger of the left hand that stands well away from its neighbor. In support of this, note how both of his index fingers stand away from their respective middle finger neighbors. Independence of thought is clearly well marked by this feature.

The basal phalanges of all of his fingers are quite developed. There is a very strong element of selfishness, which is not very helpful when he is in a social atmosphere but can be useful at awkward moments in the business arena. This is probably a developed characteristic because both heart lines are very deeply etched. The right-hand heart line is more low set than its left-hand counterpart.

Emotional and creative

Deep down, he is very emotional, warm, and considerate but doesn't trust others until he has appraised them fully. He feels things deeply and would not normally hurt a fly. He tends to get along with everyone he meets: man, woman, child, or beast, unless, of course, it is decision time. He is laid-back and little fazes him but, when he is at work or duty calls, that is different.

The percussion on both hands points toward creative curves, most prominent in the middle of the outer edges. When the curve is pronounced at the top of the palm, it shows an inspirational, creative, nature. When that at the base of the hand is more evident, there will be a practical approach. If, as in this case, it is in the middle, the owner can create and apply things practically. Phil's main interest away from work is photography.

Other Case Studies

For other case study examples, see also Anne the Cook on pages 182–185 and Alec the Engineer on pages 206–209.

TIMING EVENTS

It is not possible to forecast that on a specific day or date an event will occur, because palm reading is not that refined, nor has it ever been. The many stories of brilliant predictions allegedly from hand analysis are apocryphal and pure invention. In the East, palm reading is so inextricably linked with astrology that dating systems used by palmists are obviously astrologically based.

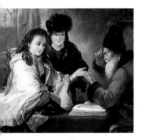

Fortuneteller

A fortuneteller reads the palm of a woman who wishes to know what the future holds for her.

Compass method

It is said that this ancient method of establishing time was used by itinerant gypsies. I have reason to doubt the authenticity of the story about the gypsies' use, but the system nevertheless often brings very good results.

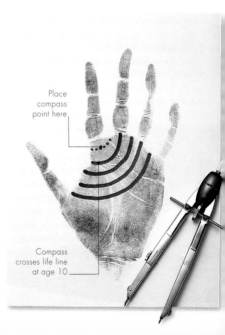

Place compass point here

Compass crosses life line at age 10

Hand Size

People new to palm reading make the same basic error and assume all hands are the same size, but they are not. Remember to allow for long or short and wide or narrow hands and for the lines on them. A long life line can stretch to the wrist in some cases, while a short line may only reach to halfway down a palm.

Age on the life line

The length of the life line is said to equal 70 years. When using the method, remember to keep questioning your subject to pinpoint accurate dates.

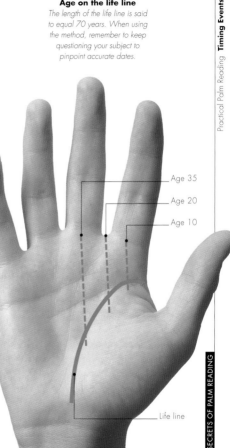

Age 35

Age 20

Age 10

Life line

Life Line Method

1 Draw an imaginary line from the middle of the bottom of the index finger straight down to the life line. Where it crosses the line of life is at approximately age ten.

2 Draw another line from between the base of the first and second fingers straight down to the life line; this intersection corresponds to age 20.

3 A third line, this time from the base of the finger of Saturn, will touch the life line at about age 35.

4 In extremely rare cases a fourth line is drawn straight from the center of the third finger, which meets the life line at about age 50.

Timing Events

Nails and timing
It is possible to time events using marks on the nails as guides.

It is possible to predict that certain events might occur but they are limited in terms of time to within a few weeks at best. Even then this information is found only on the nails. Nails take about six months to grow out so any mark on them can be measured in these terms.

A mark at the halfway point suggests an event or incident, probably the start of a period of illness, that occurred three months earlier. If the reading takes place on June 1, then the date of the incident could be anywhere between February 20 and March 10 – it's impossible to be more accurate.

However, despite all of these misgivings, there are several timing systems, all of which have some merit

attached to them. Readers are invited to experiment with what I consider to be the best and easiest to use.

The life line method

This first method (see page 191) does not allow for the size of the actual hand or how the lines may be etched but can prove to be very accurate, especially in the very early years. It would help if you began to ask questions of your subject to help pinpoint events when you ascertain each age.

After reaching age 35, the system can become unworkable. There are few people who have a life line that pushes out far enough into the palm for it to meet another line. However, in these rare cases, when this fourth line is drawn straight from the center of the third finger it meets the life line at about age 50 years.

Once these first steps have been taken, it ought to be straightforward to measure time on the rest of the life line. There are other lines on which time can be read in conjunction with this method.

The compass method

Take a pair of map dividers or an ordinary pair of compasses and place one point in the middle of the first finger at the bottom. Place the other end at the exact base of the middle finger.

Keep the first point steady on the index finger and allow the other end to swing down until it touches the life line. Where the point touches the life line is at about age ten.

Still keeping the pointer steady on the first finger, extend the divider to the base of the Apollo finger and let it swing down to the life line again. This time, it cuts through the line at about age 30.

Once again, extend the pointer to the bottom of the third finger and let it swing to the life line; this time it crosses at around age 50. Since life expectancy in ancient times was not as great as today, this was the extent of the experiment.

Older and Wiser

When these experiments were devised not many folk lived past 50, so anything beyond this ensured the person became much revered.

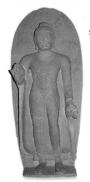

Stars and palms
In the East, dating systems used in palm reading are linked to the zodiac signs of astrology.

TIMING EVENTS
As well as using the life line and compass methods, there are other ways that can be employed to measure time using the heart, fate, and sun lines. The success of these methods depends on how strongly the lines are etched on the hand – once again the reader is invited to experiment.

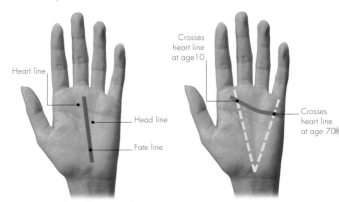

Heart line

Crosses heart line at age 10

Head line

Fate line

Crosses heart line at age 70

Time on the fate line
You can time events according to where the fate line crosses the head and heart lines.

Time on the heart line
Draw an imaginary line from the center of the base of the palm to the Jupiter and Mercury fingers.

Thread Method

1 Place one end of the thread at the life line and then lay it on the life line following every curve all the way to the end. Should the line fork, keep the thread on the stronger of the branches.

2 When you get to the end of the line, cut the thread.

3 Fold the piece of thread in half and place it again at the start of the line. When you get to the end of this doubled thread, it marks the halfway point of the life line and represents about age 36. Mark this on the hand itself.

4 Double the thread again and repeat the exercise and this time the end of the thread registers at about age 18–20. Divide this yet again and the new point is at about age 9–10.

5 Repeat this on the lower half of the line from the halfway point you marked earlier and this will help you figure out later events and date them accordingly.

Measuring curves
Lay a cotton thread along the curves of the life line, then fold the thread according to the method opposite to measure time and figure out dates.

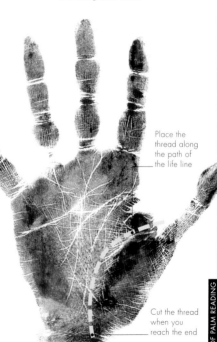

Place the thread along the path of the life line

Cut the thread when you reach the end

Timing Events

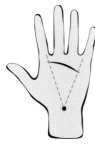

Heart line
Measuring time on the heart line was a dating method used by gypsies.

The thread method

This idea has a lot of common sense attached to it. And once again, feel free to experiment, for this too has provided highly accurate results in the past. This clever little idea involves the use of a small length of thread and a ruler – see page 195 for step-by-step details of this method.

This exercise can be successful on both the fate and sun lines because the divide and subdivide idea can give very good results. However, like the other ideas, it does not always work

for everyone. Nevertheless, if used in conjunction with the question-and-answer techniques, it can be surprising how accurately you can date events.

The fate and sun line method

You may use any of these systems on the fate line but it does not help if the line is fragmented. The best idea is to find the exact center of the base of the hand and measure to the head line as if the fate line were there in its entirety. You know it crosses the head line at age 35–36 and crosses the heart line at about 45 years.

The fate line, whether it is there or not, is divided into two between the head line and the base of the hand, the halfway point being at about age 18–20. Divide each half again for the intervening years.

The heart line method

Trace an imaginary line from the center of the base of the Jupiter finger down to the central point of the bottom of the palm. Repeat another imaginary line measuring from the base of the Mercury finger down to the same point at the bottom of the palm.

Where the line from the first finger passes over the heart line is at about age ten or so, always assuming that the heart line is physically there. In some cases the heart line can begin farther into the hand, perhaps under the finger of Saturn. Where the line from the little finger passes over the end of the heart line is reputed to be about 70 years. The mean between the two crossing points will be at about age 35–36. The divide and subdivide method may then be used to ascertain other ages.

Some modern palmists time events differently and they begin their assessments of time where the traditionalists end theirs. Once again, the reader is invited to experiment with the different methods.

Question Time

Always ask questions of your subject when using the timing methods so you can ascertain dates of certain events more accurately.

CAREER GUIDANCE

A hand reader can assess where a subject's strengths or weaknesses lie; the shape and lines of the hand can hint at the owner's potential for success in a particular career. To ascertain your subject's qualities you first need to look at the size and shape of the hand, paying particular attention to the finger set and size.

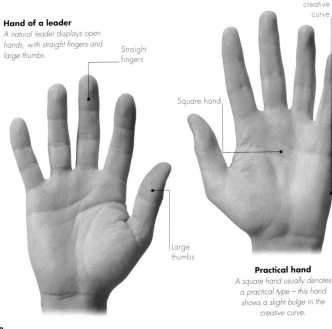

Hand of a leader
A natural leader displays open hands, with straight fingers and large thumbs.

Straight fingers

Large thumbs

Bulge in creative curve

Square hand

Practical hand
A square hand usually denotes a practical type – this hand shows a slight bulge in the creative curve.

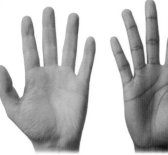

Creative hand

This is the hand of a creative person who is very sensitive and likely to be a follower. The low-set little finger indicates possible feelings of inadequacy.

Hand of a follower

These small hands are those of a follower, definitely a gofer who will do what he or she is told.

Long, round-tipped fingers

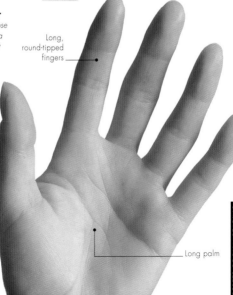

Round hand

The round hand with long palms and long fingers indicates someone who will follow a career in the creative arts.

Long palm

Career Guidance

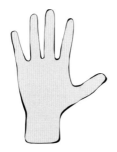

Thumb of a leader
The hands of a leader often have large, commanding thumbs.

In order to establish in which direction your subject's career lies, you must first establish the role he or she can best play – that of a leader or a follower. You must check to see if your client is a leader with supervisory or managerial talent or better suited to following instructions.

Leader

Leaders have many talents but it is the sense of power that you feel coming from them. These people often have hands that look large in comparison with their bodies. People with leadership qualities often have "open" hands, straight fingers, and large thumbs.

The thumb will almost always oppose the fingers, and a strong right-hand thumb with a weak left-hand partner is always an indication that the subject has a strong character and good personal control.

Follower

The hands of a follower are slightly smaller than usual and are often the "closed" type, with the fingers curling in toward the palm. The first finger is always shorter than the third finger and the whole hand will usually be soft to the touch.

If the little finger is low set, the subject will experience feelings of inadequacy in some way. A low-set index finger relates to lack of self-confidence and a dislike of being in the limelight. When both of these fingers are set low on the hand, there is a great deal of sensitivity – someone easily hurt by word or deed.

Practical or creative?

As we have already learned that square hands are practical, round hands are creative, and so on, we must now look at the shape. Practical people do not always make good leaders because they are conscious of the need to get a job done and they can get bogged down with the regulations.

Creative folk have many lines on their hands because their minds are never still. Unless the palm is firm to the touch with fingers longer than the palm, they are mostly concerned with the now and cannot always plan well for the future.

The small, narrow hand prefers working in the background and is often good with figures. The large wide hand prefers the open air and these people need to be free of restriction to function well, in much the same way as those with the ordinary spatulate hand.

Hand Shapes

For more information on hand shapes see pages 14–15 and 22–29.

WHICH CAREER?

Using the ideas on the previous pages for guidelines, here is a short list of careers and how to match the hand to the job – some may surprise you. These different occupations and callings all require what seem quite specific configurations but those who are successful in their various jobs do all actually have each of these shapes and markings in some way.

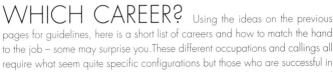

Showbusiness

An actor is likely to have a deeply curving heart line from the Jupiter mount along with a hint of a Girdle of Venus to add to his or her emotional sensitivity.

Construction

The hands of a builder will almost certainly look square and have well-developed mounts both at the top of the hand and at the bottom.

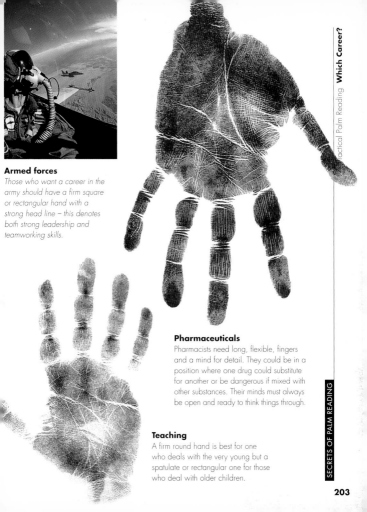

Armed forces

Those who want a career in the army should have a firm square or rectangular hand with a strong head line – this denotes both strong leadership and teamworking skills.

Pharmaceuticals

Pharmacists need long, flexible, fingers and a mind for detail. They could be in a position where one drug could substitute for another or be dangerous if mixed with other substances. Their minds must always be open and ready to think things through.

Teaching

A firm round hand is best for one who deals with the very young but a spatulate or rectangular one for those who deal with older children.

Which Career?

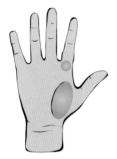

A cook's hand
A talented cook will have well-developed mounts of Jupiter and Venus.

Pharmaceuticals

Long fingers are needed due to the detailed work involved. Thumbs should be long and flexible. A long, slightly sloping head line is an advantage. The heart line must be reasonably well balanced, starting between the Saturn and Jupiter mounts and lying low in the palm.

Building work

A builder's digital mounts and base phalanges will be developed because of the sheer physical nature of the work.

The life line will be strongly etched, indicating a sound constitution – essential for withstanding the elements.

Gardening or farming

This suggests the large square or rectangular hand with knotted fingers. Practicality is needed with thoughtfulness when planning ahead. The base phalanges of each finger will be developed. The middle phalange of the Saturn finger will be longer than average, the traditional sign of the gardener or farmer. The head line should not be too long; a practical mind with some flexibility is needed for this job.

Teaching

A long first finger is essential for keeping discipline and the heart line ought to start from the mount of Jupiter and end under the Mercury mount. Which subjects suit a teacher can be seen in the head line: a long, slightly sloping line touching the top of the Luna mount would be best suited to the arts; for the science subjects, a straight line is best.

Armed forces

This is a firm square or rectangular hand with a well-balanced head line just a shade away from the life line where they start. The mounts will be strongly developed with a well-etched line of fate from wrist to palm showing the ability to give and take orders. The center of the hand, the zone of Mars, and the mouse must feel full for good health. The heart line should start on the first finger mount and it should be straight to help these people cope when promoted.

Show business

An entertainer's hand should be slightly larger than usual with a flexible thumb and long, sloping head line, ending on the top of the Luna mount. A long, straight, uninterrupted fate line from the Luna mount to the Jupiter finger will show determination and single-mindedness.

Chef or Cook

To find out what it takes to be a good cook, see the case study on Anne the Cook, pages 182–185.

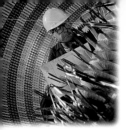

Engineering skills

A good engineer needs excellent organizational skills as well as the attention to detail required for working with complex machinery.

CASE STUDY: THE ENGINEER

Electronics is concerned mainly with the automation and instrumentation control of computers and telecommunications equipment, and both disciplines require a constantly high level of competence. Alec has been a senior production engineer for about ten years or so and his work encompasses all this type of work during the course of his duty spells.

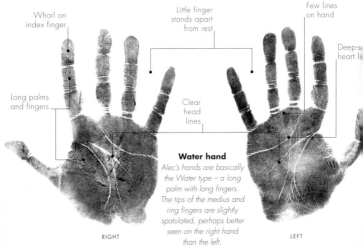

Whorl on index finger

Little finger stands apart from rest

Few lines on hand

Deep-s heart l

Long palms and fingers

Clear head lines

Water hand

Alec's hands are basically the Water type – a long palm with long fingers. The tips of the medius and ring fingers are slightly spatulated, perhaps better seen on the right hand than the left.

RIGHT

LEFT

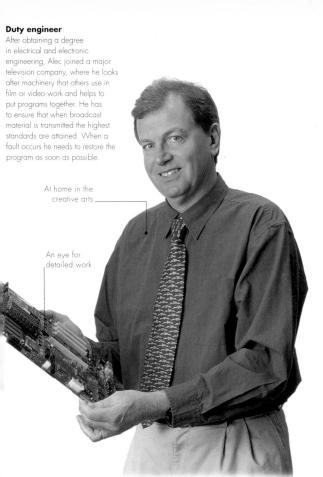

Duty engineer

After obtaining a degree in electrical and electronic engineering, Alec joined a major television company, where he looks after machinery that others use in film or video work and helps to put programs together. He has to ensure that when broadcast material is transmitted the highest standards are attained. When a fault occurs he needs to restore the program as soon as possible.

At home in the creative arts

An eye for detailed work

Alec the Engineer

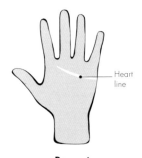

Deep set
Alec's heart line shows strong emotions and warmth – he feels things very deeply.

Heart line

Practicality and organization

Alec has to keep both feet firmly on the ground because he can become quite caught up with things. While he holds conventional views and has a few fixed opinions, the rectangular palm suggests a more extrovert nature. He will always insist that everything has a place and that there is a place for everything.

Alec is good at organizing and arranging things for and with others. It is second nature, provided he feels that it is worthwhile.

Creativity and energy

Both palms have clearly defined creative curves. The one on the left hand peaks a trifle higher than the one on the right. With such few lines on both hands they could, at a pinch, be described as "empty." He has just the four main lines and a few minor influence marks.

Both thumbs are strong and both head lines show he can concentrate for long periods. However, he knows how to relax and ease the tensions when he does finally stop and let off steam.

For the kind of detailed work with which Alec is constantly involved these hands are smaller than average. But he compensates for this with clear head lines and fairly evenly set fingers along the top of the palm that show he has plenty of self-confidence.

Those with Water hands are extremely emotionally responsive and extremely sensitive. Changes of mood, color, and atmosphere affect them, and their own moods can be predictably unpredictable.

These small, firm hands (for his size) suggest plenty of energy for anything he does get involved with but there is just a hint of a lazy streak, for both mounts of Venus are quite high and spread well into the palm.

Ambition

There is a clearly etched loop of ambition between the second and third fingers and a good loop of humor between the third and fourth fingers. Alec is ambitious and has plans for the future, showing independence, and he will not let much stand in his way, but he knows his limits.

In a family of ulnar loops on the fingertips, he has one whorl, on the right-hand index finger, which intensifies his ideals and ambitions but at times gives him a stubborn streak. Never tell him to do anything – you must ask.

Other Case Studies

For other case study examples, see Anne the Cook on pages 182–185 and Phil the Accountant on pages 186–189.

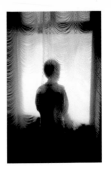

The unknown
Influence lines and special marks can give you clues to what lies ahead.

THE UNFORESEEN
No one should ever claim that they are able to foretell the future. However, a lot of people involved with the predictive arts – astrology, Tarot reading, the runes, and palm reading – can, and often do, make remarkable statements with respect to future events.

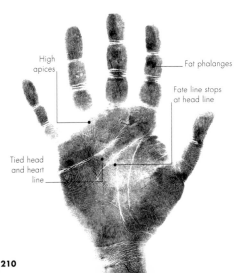

High apices

Fat phalanges

Fate line stops at head line

Tied head and heart line

Career problems
On this print the high apices show high idealism, which will interfere with any decision-making. The tied head and heart line indicates an inability to pursue a goal. The fate line stops at the head line – an indication that bad decision-making will halt a career. The fat phalanges reveal a selfish nature.

White Lines

Horizontal lines

White lines running horizontally across the first phalange of the Jupiter finger show insecurity. Possible marriage problems are highlighted if they appear on the Saturn and Apollo fingers. On the Mercury finger they indicate a communication breakdown.

Vertical lines

These may indicate hormonal imbalance. On the Jupiter finger they denote possible pituitary gland problems. On the Saturn finger they suggest a malfunction of the pineal gland. The cardiovascular system may be affected if they appear on the Apollo finger (thymus gland), while lines on the Mercury finger imply thyroid problems.

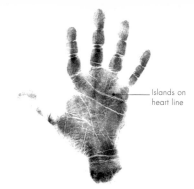

Islands on heart line

Sight or hearing difficulties

Watch out for islands on the heart line, since these warn of potential sight and hearing problems.

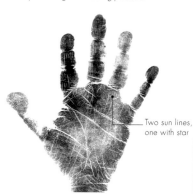

Two sun lines, one with star

Double success

Two sun lines denote two successful careers – the star emphasizes the success.

Judging Time in the Hands

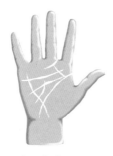

Look to the future

*Check your hands for special marks
and influence lines.*

It is simple for anyone to make a
prediction no matter what that
person's field of endeavor. After an
examination, a doctor can confidently
state that you will or will not be well
within a few days. A palmist may also
predict future events based on what he
or she has found in the hands. If the
client's character has been assessed to
within a reasonable degree, he should
also be able to predict reactions to a
given set of circumstances. If you accept
this, then you also can appreciate that
when he looks at the hands, he can scan

influence marks for matters that will
appear after the present time, interpret
them, and pronounce accordingly. This
book is packed with information on how
to do this, you just have to remember
where to look for the answers.

Predicting events

If the lines of life in both hands are
broken at the same point in time a
palmist can suggest caution, for this
implies that an accident may well occur
at that time, and a serious one at that.

If on one hand there is a square
covering the broken ends of the line, the
palmist will also say that, while the
accident is likely to occur, the subject will
recover. An emotional upset, a change
of address together with a change of
lifestyle, may be indicated.

A small line of influence running from
one of the lines of affection, the old-style
marriage lines, that merges with the
heart line is an indication of upset,
divorce, or split with the current partner.
If it is serious enough, one or both may
have to leave home to live elsewhere.

An influence line could run from the heart line at the point where the first influence line blended in and make a path to the life line. The life line may seem to weaken and not look so strong at or shortly after this point, which indicates a change of lifestyle. To try to date this we judge when the line of life receives the influence line. If you can also assess the time the influence line left the heart line it will support the theory.

You need to become reasonably proficient in judging time in the hands and fairly quickly at that. For speed, use the cotton-thread method. Base as much as you can on the life line. Cut a piece of thread and trace the line of life with it from start to finish, then cut the thread. Fold it in two, place it back on the life line from the start, and where it now ends is about age 35 or so. The rest will fall into place.

Timing Events

For more information on using the hand to time events, see pages 190–197.

FUTURE MATTERS

Do not be afraid to ask questions. Once you become proficient and learn to pick out salient points from the past, your client will want to know about future matters. These guidelines, some of which are ages old, will help pinpoint many more specific items but to list everything would take a book three or four times this size.

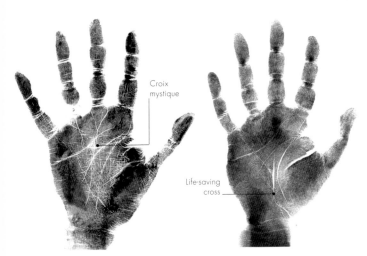

Croix
mystique

Life-saving
cross

The croix mystique

This is a clearly defined cross found beneath the middle finger between the head and heart lines and shows an interest in occult matters perhaps with healing in mind.

Life-saving cross

Normally found between the life and fate lines about 1½–2 inches (4–6cm) from the wrist. They may not actually save lives, but it shows someone who often works for the benefit of others.

Forewarned

Forewarned is forearmed. You cannot always see what lies head, so use your hand-reading skills to help you spot potential pitfalls.

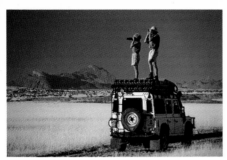

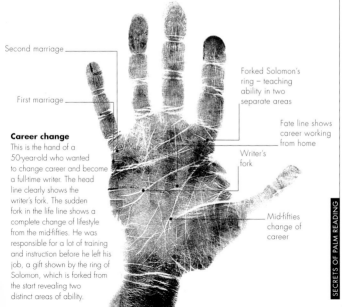

Second marriage

First marriage

Forked Solomon's ring – teaching ability in two separate areas

Fate line shows career working from home

Writer's fork

Career change

This is the hand of a 50-year-old who wanted to change career and become a full-time writer. The head line clearly shows the writer's fork. The sudden fork in the life line shows a complete change of lifestyle from the mid-fifties. He was responsible for a lot of training and instruction before he left his job, a gift shown by the ring of Solomon, which is forked from the start revealing two distinct areas of ability.

Mid-fifties change of career

Specific Marks

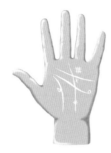

Location

Special attention should be given to where the marks are found on the hand.

Special marks must be considered in the context of where they are found. When on a line they must be dated where possible. When away from a line these marks are assessed accordingly. A mark on the thumb tip, the area of reason, may accentuate or hinder that energy.

The square of separation

A square just inside but touching the life line suggests time spent away from normal society. It could be in prison or the owner may be a monk or nun.

Stars

These marks generally emphasize incidents and wherever they are seen they intensify matters. A star on or at the end of any line always warns of impending events for good or ill. On the head line, a star shows poor decision-making or an accident to the head. On the heart line, a star usually implies emotional troubles.

A star at the end of the fate or the sun line points to a climactic success after a long period of hard work. If found on the life line, it means a potential personal injury.

A star on the first phalange of the middle finger is said to show luck through misfortune. A star on the third phalange of the third finger indicates talent and prominence by chance. A star on the third phalange of the little finger indicates spirit and eloquence.

Bars

Across any line or as horizontal marks bars always act as a hindrance. Dots are the same, but with a lesser effect.

Grilles

A grille represents a destructive force because it is a collection of lines going nowhere. Thus if found on the mount of Venus it suggests a dissipation of energy in fruitless activities. The grille always detracts from the power of a line for as long as it is there. A grille on the first finger implies possessiveness and greed. On the little finger a small grille suggests dishonesty.

Circles

These are fairly rare, but if they are seen they can be mistaken for badly formed triangles or squares when away from a line. When a circle is seen on a line it may be an island. A properly formed circle on the Apollo mount by the end of the sun line confers brilliance. Anywhere else it is an unfortunate mark.

Special Marks

For more information on special marks and their significance, see pages 92–93.

GLOSSARY

Apex The meeting point of the lines within the skin pattern.

Apollo Finger The third finger of the hand.

Arch Pattern One of the skin patterns, resembling a humpback bridge.

Bar A short influence mark, which can appear across lines or as horizontal marks denoting a hindrance.

Bracelets see **Rascettes**

Chain A series of small islands that give a chaining effect to a line.

Chirognomy The study of the basic shape of the hand.

Chiromancy The study of the lines of the hand, a traditional term.

Composite Pattern One of the skin patterns, which can be made up of a variation of an arch, loop, or whorl.

Conic Hand Traditional term, still widely used, for a round hand.

Creative Curve A clearly developed curve on the percussion (outer) side of the hand.

Croix Mystique A clearly defined cross beneath the middle finger between the head and heart lines

Cross A influence mark that may appear anywhere on a hand.

Dermatoglyphics The study of the skin patterns in the fingers and palm.

Digital Mounts The fleshy prominences under each of the four fingers.

Empty Hand A palm with few visible lines.

Family Ring A line, usually chained, that links the second and third phalange of the thumb.

Fate Line The line that starts at the wrist and goes directly to the base of the middle finger.

Full Hand A palm with a vast complexity of criss-crossing lines.

Girdle of Venus A small semicircular line or series of broken lines running from anywhere on the mount of Jupiter to the mounts of Apollo and/or Mercury.

Grille Small vertical and horizontal influence lines that form a grille pattern on the surface of the palm.

Head Line The line that begins near the line of life on the radial side of the hand and sweeps out into the palmar surface.

Health Line Another name for the Mercury line.

Heart Line The line that begins under the first finger and curves gently all the way to the percussion.

Hepatica An ancient name for the Mercury line.

Index Finger The first or Jupiter finger.

Influence Marks Small lines or patterns that can be seen anywhere on a hand.

Island A small mark on a line that suggests weakness.

Jupiter Finger The first or index finger.

Life Line This can start almost anywhere on the radial side of the hand, curving around the mount of Venus toward the wrist.

Life-saving Cross A cross touching the life and fate lines about 1½ –2 inches (4–6cm) from the wrist.

Loop Pattern One of the skin patterns – there are two types of loops: ulnar and radial.

Mars Line A line running parallel to the life line.

Medical Stigmata A small series of four or five short vertical lines slightly to the inner side of the mount of Mercury.

Medius Finger The Saturn or second finger.

Mercury Line The line that usually runs from inside the life line directly to the mount of Mercury.

Milieu Line A variation of the fate line.

Moons The small white half-moon shapes at the base of fingernails.

Mounts Fleshy prominences on the palm. There are two types: digital and palmar mounts.

Percussion The outer edge of the hand.

Phalange The section between the finger joints.

Radial The thumb or active side of the hand.

Rascettes A group of lines running across the inside of the wrist just below the palm; also known as the bracelets.

Ridges Part of the skin pattern; also horizontal or vertical marks on the nails denoting stress and strain.

Saturn Finger The second or middle finger.

Simian Line A fused head and heart line.

Square A formation of lines that may appear on the palm or fingers.

Star A starlike formation of lines that may appear on the palm or fingers.

Sydney Line A head line that completely crosses the palm.

Tented Arch One of the skin patterns that resembles a tall loop.

Tri-radius A meeting point of types of skin patterns.

Triangle A formation of lines that may appear on hands or fingers.

Ulna The outer edge of the hand; also called the percussion or instinctive side.

Via Lasciva A small horizontal or semicircular line linking the base of the Luna and Venus mounts.

Whorl One of the skin patterns, a series of concentric circles.

Zone of Mars The area of the center of the palm between the digital mounts and the tops of the Luna and Venus mounts.

FURTHER READING

There are well over 400 books available in the English language either in a secondhand or new format.

Some are a total waste of time, others are excellent. In between there are number of works that have some appeal because of an excellent dissertation on a particular theme, others because of their artwork – so often a weak point in this specialist field where one picture so easily speaks a thousand words.

These 23 books all have a special appeal for me. Many are now out of print but, should you see one in a secondhand bookstore, please buy it – it will be money well spent.

ALTMAN ROBERT *The Palmistry Workbook* Aquarian Press 1984

ASANO HACHIRO *Hands* Japan Publications 1985 (Japanese palm reading)

BASHIR MIR *The Art of Hand Analysis* Frederick Müller 1973

BEAMISH RICHARD *The Psychonomy of the Hand* Pitman 1864

BENHAM W. G. *The Laws of Scientific Handreading* Putnam 1946 (American palm reading)

CHEIRO *You and Your Hand* (Revised by Louise Owen) Jarrolds 1969

COMPTON VERA *Palmistry for Everyman* Duckworth 1952

FITZHERBERT ANDREW *Hand Psychology* Angus & Robertson 1986 (Australian palm reading)

GETTINGS FRED *The Book of the Hand* Hamlyn 1965

HARGETT J. B. *New Discoveries in Palmistry* Occident Publishing 1898 (American palm reading)

HERON-ALLEN *Manual of Cheirosophy* Ward Lock 1885 (Translated from the French)

HUTCHINSON BERYL B. *Your Life in Your Hands* Neville Spearman 1967

JACKSON DENNIS BARRY *The Modern Palmist* The World's Work 1953

JAQUIN NOEL *The Hand of Man* Faber & Faber 1938

REID LORI *Complete Book of the Hand* Pan 1991

SORELL WALTER *The Story of the Human Hand* Weidenfeld & Nicholson 1968

USEFUL ADDRESSES

SPIER JULIUS *The Hands of Children* (2nd ed.) Routledge, Kegan Paul 1955 (Translated from the German)

ST. HILL KATHERINE *The Book of the Hand* Rider 1905

TESLA PAUL *Complete Science of Hand Reading* Osiris Press 1991 (American palm reading)

WEST PETER *Life Lines* Quantum 1998

WEST PETER *Complete Illustrated Guide to Palmistry* Element Books 1998

WEST PETER *The Message of the Hands* London House 2000

WOLFF CHARLOTTE *Studies in Hand Reading* Chatto & Windus 1938

Web sites

There is a large number of sites and addresses concerned with many different facets of personality interpretation. Two of these stood out when I visited them.

Edward Campbell American author and palmist: www.edcampbell.com Extensive and frequently updated with data for the visitor to download.

Quebec Palmistry Center: www.palmistry.com Packed full of information with worldwide membership and courses on offer.

Useful Addresses

The Society for the Study of Physiological Patterns The Hon Sec, 39 Larchwood House, Baywood Square, Chigwell, Essex, IG7 4AY United Kingdom

This is the only palm reading group in the UK that correlates information between all the character assessment disciplines.

INDEX

a

actor 202, 205
affection lines 146
Air hand 26, 28, 174, 178
apices 50–53
Apollo
   finger 30
   line 138–41
   mount 52, 70, 72
areas 78, 80–81
attachment lines 148

b

back of hand 18–21
bars 216
bottom section 81
builder 202, 204
business line 132–33

c

career 198–205, 210, 215
case studies 182–89, 206–9
chirognomy 9, 12
chiromancy 12, 62
circles 217
compass method 190, 193
compatibility 180–81
conic hand 15, 19, 180–81
creative curve 71, 77
creative hand 199, 201
croix mystique 90, 214

d

dermatoglyphics 9, 12, 13
Digby Roll IV 9
digestion 168–69

e

Earth hand 23, 25, 174, 178
elementary hand 15
elements 22–9
empty hand 82, 86–87, 164–65
extroversion 166

f

family ring 150, 151, 152
farmer 204
fate line 118–25, 194, 196
fingerprints 9, 13, 42–45
fingers 30–33, 36–37
Fire hand 22, 24, 174, 178, 183, 186
flexibility 34, 164
followers 199, 200
frustration lines 146, 149
full hand 83, 84–85, 164

g

gardener 204
gesture 13, 58–61
Girdle of Venus 134–37
grilles 217

h

hand
   analysis 164–65
   exercises 162–63
   prints 46–49, 160, 161
   shape 9, 12, 14–15, 66–67, 164
   texture 68–69
hand size 16–17, 66–67, 68–69, 191
handshakes 60
handwriting 60
happiness 178–81
hard hand 69
head line 102–9
health 164, 166–73
   line 130, 131
   mount 76–77
hearing 169, 211
heart line 110–17, 194, 196–97
Hepatica 130
history 8–9

i

introversion 166
intuition line 154–57

j

Jupiter
   finger 30
   mount 52, 70, 72, 75

k

knotted fingers 32
knuckles 32–33

l

large hand 16, 68
leaders 198, 200
left-handed 16–17, 164
life line 94–101, 191, 192
life-saving cross 214
lines 64–65, 88–91, 211
liver line 130
loyalty line 151, 152
Luna mount 52–53, 70, 73

m

major lines 90–91
marks 92–93, 167, 175, 216–17
medical stigmata 157
medium hand 82, 85
Mercury
   finger 30
   line 130–33
   mount 52, 70, 72, 75
middle section 80
milieu line 121
minor lines 90–91
mixed hand 15
mounts 70–77
mouse 74, 76, 166

n

nails 35, 170–73
Neptune mount 53, 70, 73

o

origins 8–9

p

palms 50–51, 64–5
percussion side 80
pharmacist 203, 204
philosophic hand 15
Pluto mount 74, 76
practical hand 198, 201
prediction 212–13
psychic hand 15

r

radial side 80
rascettes 150, 151, 152–53
record-keeping 161
right-handed 16–17, 164
rings 54–57
   Apollo 143–5
   Mercury 143, 145
   Saturn 142–44
   Solomon 142–44
rituals 160
round hand 15

s

Saturn
   finger 30
   mount 52, 70, 72
signs 92–93
Simian line 126–28
size of hand 164
skin patterns 50–51
small hand 16, 68–69
smooth fingers 32
soft hand 69
soldier 203, 205

spacing 31, 34
spatulate hand 15, 181
square hand 14, 18, 180–81
square of separation 216
stars 216
stress 147, 149, 168
sun line 138–41, 196
Sydney line 105, 126–29

t

teacher 203, 204
thread method 195, 196
thumb 38–41
timing 190–97, 212–13
top section 81
travel lines 147, 148–49

u

unforeseen 210–11, 214–15

v

Venus mount 53, 70, 73–74, 168
Via Lasciva 134–37

w

watches 54
Water hand 27, 29, 174, 178
wealth 174–77

z

zone of Mars 74, 76
zones 79–81

ACKNOWLEDGMENTS

Special thanks go to N. J. Brown, Jill Butcher, Carla Carrington, Robert Chappell, James Cox, Julian Diamandis, Daisy Freeman, Tara Harley, R. Harrington-Lowe, Simon Harvey, S. Hodges, Ben Lacey, Jo Leitner, Kay Macmullan, Abdoulie Marong, Katharine Newton, M. Parkin, Lucrezia Pizzetti, S. Richardson, Caron Riley, Francesca Selkirk *for help with photography*

PICTURE ACKNOWLEDGMENTS

Every effort has been made to trace the copyright holders and obtain permission.
The publishers apologize for any omissions and would be pleased
to make any necessary changes at subsequent printings.

AKG, London 9, 13, 85, 145, 157, 194tl, 201. **The Bridgeman Art Library** /Simon Carter Gallery, Woodbrdige, Suffolk, UK 190cl /Galleria dell'Accademia, Florence, Italy 19tl & 197 /Gemäldegalerie, Berlin, Germany 55tl /National Gallery, London, UK 14tl & 213, 18tl /Private Collection 22tl /Vatican Museum & Galleries, Vatican City, Italy 58t. **Corbis/Bettmann** 37, 42tl, /Jacques M Chenet 59r /Ric Ergenbright 26tl /Macduff Everton 6tl /Hulton-Deutsch 55b, 59b /Wolfgang Kaehler 178tr /Leif Skoogfors 87tr. **The Image Bank** /Juan Alvarez 111tc /Georges Colbert 78tr /Romilly Lockyer 126br /Andrea Pistolesi 79t /Donata Pizzi 103tc /Alex Stewart 94b. **Tony Stone Images** 50tl, 206tl, /Martin Barraud 127tc /Christopher Bissell 170tr/Daniel Bolser 102br /Steward Cohen 186tl /Mark Douet 182tl /Dale Durfee 110b /Andrew Errington 118br /Ernst Haas 210tl /James Henry 75tl /Zigy Kalzuny 58br, 206tll /Ebby May 74tl /Martine Mouchy 74tl /Dennis O'Clair 166tl /Andreas Pollok 95tc /Alan Thornton 119tc /Art Wolfe 78bl /David Young-Wolff 215t.

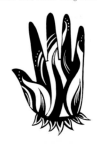